SUPERCHARGE
YOUR
IMMUNITY

SUPERCHARGE YOUR IMMUNITY

Norman D. Ford

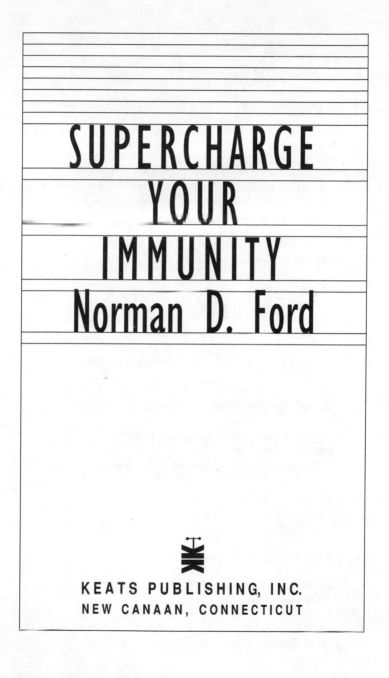

KEATS PUBLISHING, INC.
NEW CANAAN, CONNECTICUT

Supercharge Your Immunity is not intended as medical advice but solely as information and education. Please consult a medical or health professional if you have questions about your health.

SUPERCHARGE YOUR IMMUNITY
Copyright © 1998 by Norman D. Ford

Library of Congress Cataloging-in-Publication Data

Ford, Norman D., 1921–
    Supercharge your immunity / Norman D. Ford.
        p. cm.
    Includes bibliographical references and index.
    ISBN 0-87983-894-9
    1. Natural immunity.   2. Health.   3. Nutrition.   4. Exer-
cise.   I. Title.
QR185.2.F67   1998
616.07'9—dc21   97-42494
                                                          CIP

Printed in the United States of America

Keats Publishing, Inc.
27 Pine Street (Box 876)
New Canaan, Connecticut 06840-0876

Keats Publishing website address: www.keats.com

ACKNOWLEDGMENTS

In writing this book, I drew on more than 100 studies and discoveries made by top medical researchers and immunologists at many of the nation's leading medical centers. Each study was unique in that it focused on bolstering the vigor of the immune system without medical treatment or drugs. As a health reporter, my role was then to organize the best of these natural techniques into a self-care program that anyone can use to bolster his or her immunity. Many of the studies I drew on were authored by prominent researchers in the fields of immunology, cancer research, behavioral medicine and molecular and cellular biology. I regret not being able to acknowledge them all.

However, I must acknowledge my debt to the extensive research carried out by David W. Acheson, M.D., Director of Geographic Medicine and Infectious Diseases at Tufts New England Medical Center, Boston; Herbert Benson, M.D., Mindbody Medical Institute, Harvard Medical School, Cambridge, MA; Jeffrey B. Blumberg, M.D., associate director, Jean Mayer Health and Nutrition Research Center on Aging at Tufts University (also HNRC's Nutritional Immunology Lab), Somerville, MA; Joan Borysenko, Ph.D., Mindbody Health Sciences, Inc., Denver; David

Burns, M.D., associate professor of psychiatry, University of Pennsylvania School of Medicine, Philadelphia; C. Wayne Callaway, M.D. (also the Immuno-Chemistry Lab), George Washington University Medical Center, Washington, D.C.; Kenneth Cooper, M.D., Cooper Institute for Aerobics Research, Dallas; Peter Greenwald, Ph.D., director, Division of Cancer Prevention and Control, National Cancer Institute, Bethesda, MD; James Prochaska, Ph.D., Health Promotion Department, University of Rhode Island, Providence; James Rippe, M.D., director, Center for Clinical and Lifestyle Research, Shrewsbury, MA; Moshe Shiko, M.D., Director of Clinical Nutritional, Memorial Sloan Kettering Cancer Center, New York City; Stephanie Simonton, Ph.D., Behavioral Medicine Program, University of Arkansas, Little Rock, AR; David Sobel, M.D., Center for Health Sciences, Los Altos, CA.

I also drew extensively on research or studies carried out by the National Institute of Allergy and Infectious Diseases; the Diet and Cancer Branch, National Cancer Institute; the National Institute of Diabetes, Digestive and Kidney Diseases; the National Institute for Environmental Health Sciences; and the National Institute of Mental Health, all in Bethesda, MD. Also the Breast Health Center, Richmond, VA; University of Colorado Center for Human Nutrition, Denver; Duke University Medical Center, Durham, NC; Gladstone Institute of Virology and Immunology, San Francisco; Fred Hutchison Cancer Research Center, Seattle; Dana-Farber Cancer Institute, Boston; Division of Behavioral Medicine, Harvard Medical School, Cambridge, MA; Division of Immunology, Johns Hopkins School of Medicine, Baltimore; Mayo Clinic, Rochester, MN; National Institute for the Clinical Application of Behavioral Medicine, Mansfield Center, CT; National Institute of Environmental

Health Sciences, Research Triangle Park, NC; Northwest Tumor Institute, Seattle; Immunology and Rheumatology Clinic, Stanford University Hospital, Stanford, CA; Society of Behavioral Medicine, Rockville, MD; Strang Cancer Prevention Center, Harvard School of Public Health, Boston; University of Chicago Hospitals, Chicago; University of Texas M. D. Anderson Cancer Center, Houston; University of Washington Medical Center, Seattle; Weight and Eating Disorders Program, University of Pennsylvania School of Medicine, Philadelphia.

Abbreviations Used in This Book

BMI	Body Mass Index
CDC	Center for Disease Control in Atlanta
DV	Daily Value
EFA	Essential Fatty Acid
ERT	Estrogen Replacement Therapy
FDA	Food and Drug Administration
HNRC	Jean Mayer Health & Nutrition Research Center on Aging at Tufts University
IB	Immune Booster
IU	International Unit(s)
LDS	Long Slow Distance Exercise
Max	Maximum Heart Rate
mcg	Micrograms
mg	Milligrams
NIH	National Institutes of Health
NSAIDs	Nonsteroid Anti-Inflammatory Drugs
RDA	Recommended Daily Allowance
SPF	Sun Protection Factor
USDA	United States Department of Agriculture
WHR	Waist-to-Hip Ratio

CONTENTS

SUPERCHARGE
YOUR
IMMUNITY

CHAPTER ONE

Bolster Your Immunity the Whole-Person Way

How vigorous and effective is your immune system? Do you suffer from numerous colds and occasional bouts of influenza? From outbreaks of fever blisters on your lips? From persistent and chronic infections?

Do cuts and abrasions take longer than usual to heal? Have you had cancer or rheumatoid arthritis? Do you experience periods of unexplained fatigue? If you're female, are you bothered by periodic yeast infections?

A "yes" answer to one or more could indicate that the competence of your immune system may be suppressed.

But the good news is that, provided your genetic base for immunity is sound, you don't have to go on suffering from the depressing effects of weak immunity.

I

By drawing on studies from leading medical centers, researchers have developed a series of self-help strategies through which you can restore the full vigor of your immunity. Some of these techniques work on the physical level, some on the psychological level and some on the nutritional level.

In this book, I have put them all together to combine the powers of body, mind and nutrition into a single comprehensive program specifically designed to bolster immunity. In the process you can dramatically slash your risk of ever getting cancer or a serious infectious disease. And you can develop an immune system so powerful that you may easily shrug off a viral infection that would keep the average person in bed for a week.

Altogether 18 immune-enhancing techniques are described in this book. Each is called an Immune Booster (or IB for short), and each is numbered from 1 to 18. These do-it-yourself strategies embrace virtually every promising natural therapy through which you can heal and empower your immunity.

The Immune Boosters put powerful healing tools in your hands. Each IB goes beyond vitamins or drugs by allowing you to intervene naturally in the body-mind processes that suppress your immunity. Each IB improves your health and well-being. And each contains an emotional component that helps mobilize your body's healing-regeneration system.

We Can Do More to Beef Up Our Immunity Than Any Drug or Medical Treatment

The immune system — a complex organization of a trillion white blood cells plus bone marrow, antibodies and the thymus gland — defends the body from hordes of invading mi-

2

crobes whose meal of choice is human flesh. Without our immune system, we would die in 24 hours, overwhelmed by billions of lethal viruses and potential cancer cells.

How well the immune system does its job depends on whether it is weak and ineffective or vigorous and strong.

Some immunologists estimate that every day from 500 to 10,000 of our body cells are transformed into potential cancer cells. The immune system's job is to identify each of these deadly cells and to swiftly destroy it.

But in a person with weakened immunity, an occasional cancer cell is able to sneak past the immune system's defenses and to multiply into a life-threatening tumor. Thirty percent of Americans will get cancer during their lifetime, and virtually all will have a weak and depressed immune system at that time.

Another task of the immune system is to identify and destroy the millions of infectious microbes that penetrate the body each day. Besides such everyday infections as the common cold and influenza, the immune system must annihilate an army of viruses able to infect us with pneumonia, chicken pox, mumps or the peptic ulcer-causing *Helicobacter pylori* as well as hordes of bacteria capable of setting off everything from encephalitis to meningitis and a litany of strep and staph infections.

The immune system also helps to prevent, or to retard, a long list of other infections, from sexually transmitted diseases like chlamydia or gonorrhea to diphtheria, hepatitis, measles and German measles, mumps, polio, tetanus, and fungal infections like *Candida albicans.*

As it struggles to repel these and other microbial foes, the immune system constantly wages a series of cellular wars on unseen battlefields within our bodies. Almost always, the immune system triumphs over the common cold. But a person with weak immunity may take twice as long to recover as a person with a strong immune system.

A person with strong immunity is also able to annihilate many other pathogens (germs) that are not life-threatening. But medical help is usually required before even the strongest immune system can vanquish lethal diseases like encephalitis, hepatitis, meningitis or viral pneumonia.

To help beat these diseases, medical science has developed powerful monoclonal antibodies and drugs like antibiotics that directly attack the infectious disease. Yet nothing developed so far appears to significantly boost the competence of the immune system itself.

When it comes to beefing up our immunity, many immunologists believe that we ourselves can often do more to restore it to peak performance than can any doctor or medical treatment. That's because the immune system extends into almost every corner of the body-mind and it takes a whole person approach to revitalize it.

Quick Fixes Don't Always Live Up to Their Promises

While researching this book, I read several popular books on how to boost immunity. Almost without exception, their advice was to pump yourself full of vitamin and mineral supplements.

For proper function, the immune system does require a wide spectrum of vitamins and minerals. In fact, meeting the immune system's nutritional needs is one of the 18 Immune Boosters described in this book. But once our immune system's nutritional needs are met, taking additional megadoses of vitamins rarely helps.

I found equally misleading claims in several other books that extolled the virtues of a single nutrient—often a hormone that is claimed to boost serotonin levels. Whether it was blue-green algae, co-enzyme Q10, DHEA, melatonin, royal jelly, shark cartilage or whatever supplement is currently being hyped, a single magic bullet is rarely able to boost immunity to any extent.

Certainly, each of these nutrients may have limited benefits for one or two ailments or dysfunctions. But none is a universal panacea, and some may have detrimental side effects. For example, by raising male testosterone levels, DHEA can increase the risk of prostate cancer.

When I wrote my first health book years ago, the editor cautioned that any mention of exercise or willpower would ruin sales. If you read many health books today, you know that most authors still follow this advice. A book that tells how to send your immunity soaring by popping a few pills makes convincing reading for those who are gullible—and even better advertising copy.

The trouble with these books is that they cover only a tiny portion of the topic. Taking nutritional supplements totals less than 5 percent of the total number of steps you can take to upgrade your immunity. Yet most authors choose to ignore the other 95 percent.

So Move Over Magic Bullets

The Immune Boosters in this book are strictly no-nonsense techniques that really work. To get you started, several techniques are actually quick fixes in that they are simple and easy to do. Immune Booster #15, in fact, is one of the most powerful immune enhancers. Medical studies have proved

5

that it can raise your immuno-competence by an appreciable amount in just 30 minutes. And IB #13 simply requires you to get an extra hour of sleep each night.

These are easy techniques that require little effort. IBs #1, #2 and #3 are equally simple.

But the real heavyweights—the IBs that make you almost cancer-proof and that dramatically slash your risk of ever coming down with an infectious disease—may require a little more effort and time.

Actually, all the Immune Boosters are based on *action therapy*. That is, they require you to use your mind and muscles to do what it takes to succeed in revving up your immunity. Action therapy requires you to take an active role in rejuvenating your immune system, and it's a hundred times more powerful than passively sitting on a couch while you pop a pill and watch TV.

This book is also based on a series of recent scientific discoveries so astounding that they stand our earlier knowledge of immunity on its ear. When I put together the many findings from a score of leading research centers, this is the overall picture that emerged.

The Immune System Exactly Mirrors Our Mood and Self-Esteem

Immunologists at the National Institutes of Health and elsewhere have discovered that the competence of our immune system exactly mirrors our mood and emotions and the way we feel about our body and health.

Positive thoughts and feelings enhance immuno-competence, while negative thoughts and emotions suppress and weaken the vigor of our immunity. To a great extent, our thoughts and feelings can make us sick or make us well. The immune system responds immediately to our mood and to how our body looks and feels. For instance, being and looking 20 percent overweight can significantly depress our immuno-competence. So can doing any of the health-destroying things listed below.

Our Immune System Will Supercharge Itself If We Stop Doing Things That Weaken and Suppress It

For many of us, the problem is not so much to beef up our immunity as to stop eating and doing things that weaken the immunity we already have. Some of the principal causes of immuno-suppression include:

Smoking
Unresolved emotional stress
Feeling depressed, anxious, hopeless or helpless
Overloading the immune system with too many cancer cells
    or microbial infections
Sedentary living and failing to exercise
Being 20 pounds or more overweight
Eating a high-fat diet containing too few fruits, vegetables
    and whole grains
Excessive sunbathing
Insufficient sleep
A nutritional deficiency or malnutrition
Taking immuno-suppressive or certain other drugs, includ-
    ing recreational drugs
Pushing oneself to the physical limit for too long
Consuming more than two alcoholic drinks per day if you're
    male and more than one drink if you're female

7

Medical procedures such as surgery or radiation
Failing to breast-feed babies

In infants and small children—especially those not breast-fed—the immune system is immature and has difficulty fighting off an array of familiar childhood infections. But by puberty, the immune system has memorized the antigens (recognition codes) of many common viral and bacterial diseases. The immune system in a healthy 14-year-old is already supercharged.

One reason is that most cancer cells take years to develop and the average young person is generally free of proliferating cancer cells. Destroying hundreds or thousands of freshly activated cancer cells each day is a frequent cause of immune system overload in people 45 and over.

Provided a 14-year-old is physically active, not overweight and avoids cigarettes, drugs and the worst of the nutritional disasters in which teenagers tend to indulge, his immune system is able to defend the body against a wide range of diseases and dysfunctions.

Each year thereafter in a healthy person, the immune system gradually loses some of its vigor. Even then, provided we avoid the counterproductive habits just listed and remain slender and active, our immune system can continue to defend us effectively into our 80s and 90s or to age 100 and beyond.

By contrast, a person who indulges in several of the immune-suppressing habits just listed often experiences a rapid decline in immunity. By middle age, her immune system is often so weakened that it can no longer protect the body. Cancer cells are able to survive and clone into a tumor while pneumonia or other infections often prove fatal.

But this doesn't have to happen.

Even if your health isn't perfect, chances are good that you can restore your immunity to the optimal level for your age in just a short time. The way to do it, of course, is to adopt and practice some or all of the Immune Boosters described in this book.

That's because the Immune Boosters force you to stop making the poor health choices that send your immunity reeling. Instead, they steer you toward wise health choices that sending your immunity soaring

The Power of Our Immune System Is Under Our Direct Personal Control

Having a strong immune system is not just a matter of good genes or good luck. For example, a cancerous tumor usually occurs only when our immune system is weakened or suppressed. According to the National Cancer Institute, at least 80 percent of all cancers are caused by the same immune-suppressing habits listed in the previous section.

Each of these immune-destroying habits—from sedentary living to being overweight to eating a high-fat diet or not getting enough sleep—are all things over which we have direct personal control.

Each of us has it within our power to stop abusing our immune system with fat-laden foods and to switch instead to a diet rich in cancer-fighting fruits and vegetables. By forcing us to make other wise health choices, the Immune Boosters give us almost total control over the potency of our immune system.

By making the Immune Boosters a permanent part of our lifestyle, we can boost our immunity to the point where our risk of getting cancer is 50 to 75 percent less than that of the average American. (The actual percentage depends on the type of cancer; 90 percent of the risk of lung cancer can be prevented.)

We can also dramatically reduce the risk of ever getting a serious infectious disease, including some allergies and certain autoimmune diseases like rheumatoid arthritis. And though cardiovascular diseases are not directly related to immunity, we can also slash our risk of ever getting a heart attack or stroke.

How We Can Stop Overloading Our Immune System

Activated cancer cells can overload the immune system if too many develop at the same time or if one or more forms a tumor. Each time the immune system has to expend its energy and resources to destroy a cancer cell, its ability to destroy more cancer cells or microbes is significantly diminished.

Yet every day most people over 45 seriously weaken their immune systems by producing hundreds or thousands of fresh cancer cells.

Obviously, the fewer activated cancer cells we have in our bodies, the less they can overload and weaken our immune systems. Now it may be difficult to believe this. But each of us has a great deal of personal control over the number of activated cancer cells that our bodies produce. *We each have it within our personal control to prevent activation of between 50 and 80 percent of the potential cancer cells that form in our bodies each day.*

How? Cigarette smoking, failing to exercise, being overweight and eating a high-fat diet are all ways that increase the number of cancer cells that our bodies produce. *But new research has proven that by eating more foods each day that grow on plants, we can significantly prevent most types of cancer, and we may even retard the growth of certain tumors that already exist.*

THE REAL ROLE OF NUTRITION

Nutrition plays a key role in rejuvenating immunity but not in the way that most of us expect. While nutritional supplements can prevent vitamin and mineral deficiencies, it is micronutrients in fruits and vegetables that really free our immune system from chronic overload.

It works like this.

Scores of major studies have implicated meat, poultry, fried foods, eggs, all dairy foods but nonfat and polyunsaturated cooking oils, together with hydrogenated vegetable oils, as prime causes of most cancers.

These foods have several things in common. None has any appreciable fiber. All are powerful promoters of free radicals. And they contain almost no antioxidants or anticarcinogens.

Free radicals are electrically charged molecules formed when dietary fat is oxidized in the body. These rogue molecules then roam through the body, causing rapid aging and playing havoc with the body to where, in some cells, cancer is activated. The more foods we eat that promote free radicals, the more activated cancer cells the body produces.

Antioxidants are molecules that neutralize free radicals and disarm them. Antioxidants are found primarily in plant foods that grow in sunlight. The more plant foods we consume, the less chance there is that free radicals will activate cancer in our body.

Additionally, just about all foods that grow on plants also

11

abound with anticarcinogens (chemicals that fight cancer). Thus the more vegetables, fruits, whole grains, legumes, nuts and seeds that we eat—and the fewer foods that promote free radicals—the less chance there is of immune system overload. At the same time, our risk of ever getting cancer is dramatically reduced.

IB #4 describes a dozen powerful micronutrients found only in plant foods, each of which can prevent cancer or slow or block the cancer process. These micronutrients are so powerful that even in smokers, eating five or more servings of fruits and vegetables each day halves the risk of developing lung cancer.

While some nutritional supplements such as vitamin C or E are believed to be antioxidants, when it comes to boosting our immunity the real superstars are foods that grow on plants. Micronutrients in plant foods provide tremendous health benefits. They can prevent blood clots and heart attacks and slow the aging process, and some are able to block angiogenesis or the development of blood vessels in growing tumors. Without a blood supply, a malignant tumor cannot thrive.

Plant Foods Are Strong Medicine for the Immune System

Until recently, it was thought that a single vitamin or a single nutrient with antioxidant properties could prevent cancer. But in a series of major studies, single nutrients such as beta-carotene proved disappointing.

Now researchers believe that instead of taking a few single nutrients in supplement form, we should eat a variety of plant-based foods, each of which contains a complex array of antioxidants and anticarcinogens.

When we eat a variety of fruits, vegetables, whole grains, legumes, nuts and seeds, these micronutrients work together to prevent or retard the cancer process. Certainly some single nutrients such as vitamins C or E appear to have antioxidant properties. But they can never replace the complex power of antioxidants and anticarcinogens in plant foods.

Literally hundreds of studies have supported these findings. Several of the largest studies have implicated fat, meat and fried foods as a prime cause of cancer. In the large-scale Nurses' Health Study, women who ate the most animal fat were twice as likely to develop cancer as women with a lower intake.

Another study of cancer mortality in 40 nations by Gerhardt N. Schrauzer, Ph.D. found that breast and intestinal cancer were most common in nations with the highest intake of meat and fat and lowest in nations with the highest intake of plant foods.

Even as this was being written, a fresh study released by Harvard Medical School confirmed that most cancers were caused by just three factors: smoking, lack of exercise and a poor diet (meaning the standard high-fat American diet that contains almost zero fruits or vegetables). Each of these causes is under our direct, personal control. Only 2 percent of cancers appeared to be caused by toxins in the environment.

While medical officials say that almost one American in three will get cancer at some time in life, they fail to point out that most cancers are eminently preventable. By adopting all or some of the Immune Boosters in this book, we can dramatically lower our risk of ever getting cancer. In the process, we can free our immune system from cancer overload and allow it to regain its natural vigor.

SLASH YOUR RISK OF CATCHING COLDS AND OTHER INFECTIONS

Every day millions of viruses, bacteria and fungi penetrate the body, and many are able to cause serious diseases.

Pneumonia, for example, can be carried by either a virus or a bacterium. In either case, it enters through the mouth or nose. Most pneumonia microbes are blocked by tiny cilia hairs in the nose or are repelled by saliva. But occasionally a microbe makes it to the lungs. Once there the microbe multiplies at an explosive rate.

However, the pathogen is quickly recognized by patrolling immune cells. Swiftly, the entire immune response is turned on, and billions of immune cells begin to manufacture antibodies (protein molecules that can disable a virus or bacterium). But that may take several days.

Meanwhile, the struggle between the immune system and pneumonia clogs the 300 million tiny air sacs in the lungs. Blood pressure plummets, and breathing becomes difficult and shallow. In a day or two, the victim can barely inhale sufficient oxygen to stay alive.

In elderly people or infants, or in anyone whose immune system is already weakened by overload, lung congestion can become so severe that the liver and kidneys may fail. When that happens, immune cells begin to die from lack of oxygen, leaving the pneumonia microbes free to spread throughout the body.

Antibiotics can kill bacterial pneumonia. But when the immune system is already overloaded by having to destroy more cancer cells or other microbes than it can handle, viral pneumonia is often fatal. As the sixth leading cause of death in the United States, pneumonia afflicts 4 million people annually and kills 76,000.

Like many other infections, pneumonia usually becomes life threatening when the immune system is overburdened and weakened by having to kill too many proliferating cancer cells and more infectious microbes than it can deal with at one time.

But just as we ourselves can help reduce the proliferation of cancer cells, so we can help to slash the number of infectious microbes that enter the body. For instance, if you seem to catch everything that's going around, you can halve your risk of getting a cold or influenza simply by refraining from touching your nose or mouth with your fingers.

That's just one of many simple, natural techniques through which you can exert positive control over the number of microbes that penetrate your body. They're all described in IB #11, and using them can help you reduce much of the overload that may be crippling your immunity.

Keep Your Inoculations Up-to-Date

Another way to amplify your immunity is to keep your inoculations up-to-date. Vaccinations may not seem entirely natural, and you may have a slightly sore arm or a minor reaction for a day afterward. But killed or weakened microbes are used in all vaccines, and the amount is far too small to overload the immune system.

The amount used is just enough to impress the antigen of that disease on the immune system's memory cells. Should the disease itself then penetrate the body, immune cells carrying its antigen in their memory can swiftly identify the intruder and trigger a bodywide immune response. Almost invariably then, the immune system is able to squelch the disease before it can begin.

Among common diseases for which vaccines are available

15

are chicken pox, diphtheria, German measles or rubella, hepatitis A and B, influenza, measles, meningitis, mumps, pertussis or whooping cough, polio, rabies (if bitten), and tetanus.

Being vaccinated against one of these diseases places a thousand times less burden on the immune system than having the disease itself. Being vaccinated could also save your life or that of your child.

THE DEVASTATING EFFECTS OF EMOTIONAL STRESS

Abundant evidence exists to prove that after cigarette smoking, emotional stress is the most powerful single suppressor of immunity. Unresolved emotional stress stimulates secretion of adrenal hormones such as cortisol that directly inhibit immune function. Studies show that millions of Americans experience severe stress several times each week while others are stressed out permanently.

Once stress suppresses immunity, opportunistic diseases such as cancer or infections are able to survive. Almost always, people who live under stress experience frequent colds and other infections and eventually cancer or heart disease.

For example, several years ago a Northwest National Life Insurance study found that 50 percent of workers in high-stress jobs had frequent colds, bronchitis and pneumonia. Another study at UCLA concluded that people with a history of job stress had a risk of developing colon or rectal cancers five times greater than the general public.

Oncologists (cancer specialists) have also noted that cancer is most likely to appear after a period of prolonged stress such as an angry divorce, death of a spouse, a financial loss

16

or unemployment. Prolonged stress may also lead to anxiety, depression, helplessness, and hopelessness, each a potent suppressor of immunity.

Don't Let Stress Sabotage Your Immunity

Actually, most stress is caused not by a potentially stressful life event but by the way we perceive it. Smith and Jones both work on an automobile production line. When production is automated, the workforce is downsized, and both lose their jobs.

Smith perceives his unemployment as a catastrophe. He sees no alternative source of employment and believes he will lose his home, furniture and car. Soon Smith experiences such common stress symptoms as tight shoulders and muscle tension, anxiety and depression, and he begins to suffer from frequent colds and infections.

Jones, on the other hand, perceives his unemployment as a welcome release from a tedious job and a wonderful opportunity to train for a new and rewarding career. Jones feels buoyant and invigorated and bounces out of bed each morning feeling fit and optimistic.

Both men faced exactly the same potentially stressful life event. It wasn't the unemployment itself that was stressful. It was the way Smith perceived it that created his stress. The stress occurred inside Smith's mind. And he created it all by perceiving the world through a filter of negative and inappropriate beliefs.

You don't have to become another Smith.

IB #18 describes a series of simple action steps through which you can take charge of your personality and replace negative beliefs with positive beliefs. The immediate result is to

17

transform immune-suppressing stress into immune-enhancing relaxation. And if you're willing to do what it takes to succeed, you can transform depression into optimism with a proven technique called *cognitive training*.

Fewer Pounds Strengthen Immunity

Being 20 pounds or more overweight is another common way to suppress immunity. For most Americans, shedding weight is a losing battle. But IB #5 proves that almost all of us can take control of our weight, provided we're willing to do what it takes to succeed.

Based on revolutionary new findings at the Jean Mayer USDA Human Nutrition Research Center, IB #5 demonstrates that being overweight is not the problem. The real problem is a dysfunction in the shape and composition of our bodies.

Due to these discoveries, as of January 1, 1996, the USDA discarded its ideal weight tables and introduced a new measurement of body health called *body mass index* (BMI). BMI measures the ratio between your body's lean muscle mass and your body fat.

IB #5 shows how to calculate your BMI in two minutes. Most people have a BMI between 20 and 35+. A BMI over 25 indicates a loss of muscle and a gain in body fat. A BMI of 27 or more indicates poor body composition due to too much fat and too little muscle, while a BMI over 30 is what most of us know as obesity. The higher your BMI, the more muscle you have lost and the more your immunity is likely to be suppressed.

Instead of double talk about dieting and cutting calories, IB #5 defines overweight as a dysfunction in the shape and composition of the body due to loss of skeletal muscle through lack of exercise. Each year after age 20, the average sedentary person loses half a pound of muscle. By age 40, most Americans have lost 10 pounds of muscle.

Since muscle burns calories 24 hours a day while fat burns almost none, this translates in the average person into a weight gain of 1 pound every 11 days—almost all of it in fat. (If we don't actually gain weight that fast, it's because we're burning off some of our excess calories through physical activity.)

It's no wonder Americans can't lose weight!

But here again the solution is under our direct, personal control. Instead of dieting to lose fat, we need to exercise to restore the muscle mass we have lost. As we do, the shape and composition of our body will improve. Our basic metabolism will rise, and we will begin to gradually burn off our excess fat.

As you read through this book you will discover that there's a natural antidote to almost everything that suppresses our immunity. When we add it all up, it lies within the direct personal control of each of us to adopt and make these antidotes a permanent part of our lifestyle. The payoff is a powerful immune system and an almost lifelong freedom from cancer and most infections.

Can Drugs Help Your Immunity?

When this book was written, medical treatment could do relatively little to boost your immune power. Recent developments like bone marrow transplants and monoclonal antibodies could help in some cases. But most drugs actually suppress immunity rather than empower it.

By destroying fungi and bacteria, antibiotics give a powerful assist to an immune system already overwhelmed by invading microbes. But antibiotics don't increase immuno-competence. Nor can they kill viruses. Rather than beefing up immunity, most drugs are used to combat diseases that the immune system fails to halt.

I'd like to emphasize here that nothing in this book is intended to discourage you from seeing a doctor or taking medication. The Immune Boosters in this book are designed to complement medical treatment, not to challenge it. In fact, if you have any symptom of cancer or any type of infection that does not clear up in a few days, I strongly urge you to see a doctor. You don't normally need to consult a physician for a cold or influenza, but if complications develop, these minor infections could lead to life-threatening pneumonia.

Obviously, some diseases require medical treatment and drugs. But all too often we resort to tranquilizers, antidepressants and diet drugs to help beat lifestyle problems like feeling stressed, experiencing a downer or being overweight. Stress, depression and obesity are all immuno-suppressants. But each can also be easily remedied by using the natural IBs in this book.

Tranquilizers, antidepressants and diet drugs can only do what a healthy body-mind can do for itself. They're a great help for people who are unwilling or unable to help themselves. But several IBs in this book describe natural techniques that achieve far better results without drugs.

Most drugs are not a simple panacea. Many have side effects so unpleasant that up to one-third of patients stop taking their medications. Many drugs are expensive. A sizable number fail to work. And some create new diseases that weren't there before.

Here, to help you evaluate them, is a brief rundown of drugs associated with the causes, or the results, of immuno-suppression.

Diet Drugs Are Not Miracle Cures

If your BMI is over 25—or if you're overweight—one way to help your immunity is to restore your body composition to normal. One person in three in America is seriously overweight and the problem is so widespread that obesity is now considered a chronic disease. Physicians define obesity in men as having 25 percent or more body weight in fat; for women, the figure is 30 percent.

Since most people are unwilling to exercise, millions are turning to diet drugs. The drugs work by suppressing appetite. But they are successful only when taken in conjunction with exercise and a low-fat diet. When this book was written, the drugs were recommended only for people 20 percent or more overweight (that is, for anyone with a BMI of 30 or over).

The drugs don't work for everyone. In a test of 900 users of a leading diet drug, in which participants also exercised and followed a low-fat diet, only 37 percent lost more than 10 percent of their original weight, and only 21 percent lost more than 15 percent of their weight. In some people, the drugs may also cause changes in short-term memory, diarrhea, disturbed moods and sleep patterns, drowsiness and dry mouth, most of which disappear in time.

Moreover, the drugs work only when taken. Weight shoots back up immediately when they are stopped. Few people can maintain the weight loss unless they take the drugs for life. Overall, results are hardly dramatic. New and better

21

drugs may be developed one day. But when this book was written, most diet drugs were ineffective unless used in conjunction with aerobic and strength-building exercise and a low-fat, largely plant-based diet.

On the plus side, for people with morbid obesity, the drugs can help lower the risk of cancer, heart disease and immuno-suppression, and they can give a boost to immunity by decreasing depression and raising self-esteem. Yet anyone can get the same results without the drugs by simply using Immune Boosters #5, #6 and #8.

Sobering Facts About Antidepressants

Few people take anti-depressant medication to bolster their immunity, but depression is one of several negative emotions which can devastate immunocompetence. By alleviating depression in roughly two-thirds of people who take them, antidepressant medications do help rejuvenate immunity. But the drugs work only by masking symptoms, and to date, none is able to reverse the underlying condition.

Approximately one-third of people are not helped by these drugs, or they experience such side effects as anxiety, diarrhea, drowsiness, drug-induced agitation, dry mouth, headache, inhibited sex function, insomnia, loss of appetite, loss of libido, nausea and skin rash. Pregnant women who have continued taking certain antidepressants into their third trimester have also been more likely to give birth prematurely or to have babies with minor birth defects.

For those willing to use their minds and muscles to do what it takes to succeed, IBs #15, #16 and #18 can achieve far superior results without these medications.

Immune-Suppressing Drugs Assault Our Immunity

Powerful immune-suppressing drugs are used to inhibit the immune system so that it will not reject an organ transplanted from another person. They may also be used to treat severe cases of rheumatoid arthritis, a disease in which, instead of defending the body, the immune system attacks the body's own cells.

In either case, immune-suppressing drugs significantly increase risk of cancer and infections, and they may also damage the liver and kidneys. One day, less damaging drugs may appear. Meanwhile, anyone treated with immune-suppressing drugs should realize that they do indeed suppress imunity, and they must usually be taken regularly for the rest of one's life.

Corticosteroids are a group of natural hormones produced by the adrenal glands. They are also powerful immunosuppressants. People call them *stress hormones* because the adrenals secrete corticosteroids when under stress. This is one way in which stress suppresses immunity.

When all else fails, corticosteroids may also be used to prevent an allergic reaction by the immune system. To many people, suppressing their immunity seems a heavy price to pay for relief from an allergy. If you agree, look up IB#14 and see if there isn't a natural alternative.

PREVENTING CANCER IS EASIER THAN CURING IT WITH DRUGS

According to the National Cancer Institute, since 1975 incidence of cancer has risen 18.6 percent in men and 12.4

23

percent in women due primarily to huge increases in cancer of the breast, lung and prostate. Certainly, fewer people die of cancer nowadays. But despite advances in medical treatment, most cancer therapy still follows a "slash and burn" philosophy.

Today's chemo drugs are less harsh, but cancer cells often develop a resistance to these drugs. Called *multiple drug resistance receptor*, the mechanism expels chemo drugs from cells as rapidly as they enter.

Although prostate cancer is one of the most easily preventable forms of the disease, millions of men still receive radiation and hormone treatment for this disease. Treatment may still result in dampened sexuality and may not prevent the cancer from spreading into the lung or brain and forming another tumor.

None of our Immune Boosters claims to be a cure for cancer, but most can certainly help prevent it. Some fruits and vegetables may also contain micronutrients that inhibit further tumor growth. Certainly, if you have any symptoms of cancer, you should see a doctor immediately. The seven primary symptoms of cancer are a change in bowel or bladder habits, a change in a mole or wart, indigestion or difficulty in swallowing, a lump in the breast, a nonhealing sore, a persistant cough or hoarseness and unusual bleeding.

Otherwise, by adopting IBs #3, #4 and #8, you may very well make yourself as cancer-proof as it is possible to become. This is true even if you have already had cancer and been cured. By adopting these IBs—with your doctor's permission, of course—you can significantly decrease the chance that your cancer will return.

EXOTIC NEW MICROBES ARE SWEEPING THE WORLD

Until a few years ago, immunologists mainly focused on heating cancer. But as destruction of the rain forests and construction of huge dams force microbes to relocate, deadly viruses and bacteria are mutating across the world, sweeping the globe with new epidemics that have already decimated populations in a dozen African countries.

America hasn't escaped. Few of us may have noticed, but between 1980 and 1992, infectious diseases rose from being the fifth killer of Americans to being third. It's partly due to overuse of antibiotics. From 1980 to 1992, hospital-caused infections rose by 36 percent. Yet fresh hordes of killer microbes are brought to our shores daily by commercial jets.

As these serial killers learn new survival techniques, infections we once thought were licked have resurfaced in full force. Drug-resistant TB has staged a comeback in several U.S. states while cases of cholera, gonorrhea, hepatitis A and B, pneumonia, respiratory tract infections and septicemia—a potentially fatal blood bacteria—are soaring in many countries. All are more common than HIV.

New drug-resistant strains of bacterial meningitis, bubonic plague, cholera, dengue fever, TB, yellow fever and other diseases once thought eliminated are reappearing across the globe. Meanwhile, new and unrecognizable infectious diseases show up frequently in U.S. hospitals, particularly foodborne illnesses. Many are resistant to every antibiotic that currently exists. And new antibiotics may not be developed for years.

Researchers at the Center for Disease Control (CDC) and elsewhere have cautioned that even the most powerful drugs

25

may not save us from the infectious diseases of the future. Modern bacteria have learned to exchange genes with similar life forms, and they can multiply so rapidly that within weeks, new strains can appear that are resistant to the latest antibiotics and other drugs.

But one thing *is* certain. When disease hits, people with stronger immune systems always fare better. And when it comes to dealing with diseases of the future—a future that may be only a few years away—we may well need all the immuno-competence we can summon.

Global Warming Helps Deadly Microbes Spread

At the same time, global warming is powering the spread of malaria and yellow fever toward the southern United States. Within a few years, U.S. populations living close to the Mexican border may be at risk for diseases we thought were wiped out a century ago.

Viruses are sneaky and can change the antigen on their outer surface to escape detection by immune system cells. In his 1996 book, *The Sixth Extinction*, paleoanthropologist Richard Leakey describes how the worldwide decline in environmental quality could produce a crop of entirely new microbes with the potential to wipe out half the human race.

So great has been the spread of contagious diseases that many doctors are now specializing in infectious diseases. Meanwhile, the CDC has cautioned physicians to go slow on using antibiotics. Unnerving messages are coming from immunologists across the country, warning that the rise of antibiotic-resistant microbes could threaten the survival of anyone with compromised immunity.

New Plagues Are a Chilling Possibility

As routine vaccination programs are interrupted by poverty and wars, public health officials everywhere are concerned that a new plague could sweep the world. A plague can occur only when there is no immunological memory of the microbe's antigen in the human population. All it would take to wipe out half the human race is an absolutely new microbe with an antigen so different that it might not be recognized by anyone's immune system.

The Ebola virus came perilously close to meeting these requirements. The chance that another, even more deadly mutation could occur at any time is quite high. A brand new microbe unrecognized by any human immune system would meet little resistance. Before our immune systems could fight back, several billion people could be dead.

It's no secret that some officials at the CDC believe that a new pandemic of influenza will eventually sweep the world. An entirely new strain could wipe out far more than the 20 million who died in the pandemic of 1918. Infectious disease prevention programs are underfunded worldwide, including in the United States, while many Third World countries have no public health infrastructure at all.

A strong immune system may not save us entirely. But if any plagues come my way, I'd sooner have a scrappy immune system ready to fight back than one weakened by all the vicissitudes of modern living.

MIND OVER IMMUNITY

Much of our immune system operates on a nonphysical level. Thus our feelings and emotions can often do more to

27

raise or lower our immuno-competence than any chemical or mechanical cause. As a result, many immunologists are convinced that the immune system cannot be upgraded by a pharmacist but only by the body-mind itself.

How the Immune System Spearheads Our Healing-Regeneration System

Perhaps the immune system's most important task is its role as the core component of our healing-regeneration mechanism. Supporting the immune system, and boosting its immuno-competence, is a series of powerful psychological components known as *effects*.

These include the placebo, enabling, endorphin and knowledge effects. All are highly subjective and function only as beliefs and emotions. Yet each works synergistically to reinforce the others.

Only the immune system is physical. The four effects work on a very subtle level. Yet they rank among the most powerful immune boosters in existence. Together, they are responsible for most cases of healing or disease reversal and remission.

The literature is filled with case histories of people who have experienced spontaneous recoveries from illnesses deemed terminal. And rare cases have occurred in which large, malignant tumors have regressed and disappeared without medical treatment. When researchers investigated, they found that in every case recovery was preceded by a sudden change to a strongly positive mind-set that sent immunity soaring.

The powers of belief, faith, hope and suggestion have a tremendous effect on immunity. A strong belief is often a more powerful healer than many drugs. And the immune system is almost totally responsive to the placebo and other psychological effects that comprise our healing-regeneration system.

Each time we use one of the Immune Booster techniques, we set in motion an emotional component that unlocks our healing regeneration system.

The Awesome Healing Power of the Placebo Effect

The placebo effect is an immune-boosting mechanism in the mind that arises from a person's faith, belief and expectation in the healing power of a therapy rather than from the therapy itself. Studies show that the placebo effect can improve a person's chances of recovery from almost any nonfatal disease or injury—including surgery—by an average of 33 percent.

For example, most patients who believe strongly that they will recover are up and around after surgery in one-third less time than those with weaker beliefs.

For centuries, witch doctors and shamans have known that the remedy they used was less important than the attitude they could arouse in the patient. Through much of human history, these native healers have used rituals and symbols like animal sacrifices, rattles and wooden masks to trigger the placebo effect in people who were sick.

Recent research suggests that although the rituals and symbols have changed, approximately one-third of the benefit derived from modern drugs and medical treatment still arises from the placebo effect. For millions of Americans, the hospital room has become the temple of healing, the doctor in his white coat is the high priest and the bottle of pills is the modern-day symbol of healing.

Whenever a drug is given a clinical test, the action of the placebo effect must be added to the action of the drug in assessing results. In many trials, especially on people with disorders related to the immune system, tests have shown that the placebo effect often provides greater benefit than the drug's pharmaceutical action.

We can put the placebo effect to work immediately by developing a strong faith and belief in the power of the Immune Booster techniques we are using. This will enhance their immune-boosting power by up to 33 percent. Then by using other psychological healing mechanisms—such as the enabling or endorphin effect—we can magnify the benefits of the placebo effect. Each time we expand the power of the placebo effect, we give a huge boost to our immuno-competence.

Empowering Your Immunity with the Enabling Effect

The enabling effect is the psychologists' term for the empowerment we experience whenever we attribute an improvement in our health to our own efforts rather than to a passive therapy such as a drug or medical treatment. A passive therapy is when something is given to us, or done to us, by someone else while we passively do nothing.

This rarely happens when we use an Immune Booster because almost every one is an active therapy that requires us to take an active role in upgrading our health.

As we begin to use an Immune Booster and watch it succeed, we naturally attribute each success to our own efforts. Doing so empowers us with formidable amounts of enabling effect.

The secret to mobilizing the enabling effect is to provide

ourselves with constant feedback. Once we begin using an IB and maybe our weight is dropping as we eat more and more fruits and vegetables and fewer foods that promote free radicals, that's all the feedback most of us need to keep our enabling effect turned on at full strength.

If you wish to harness the power of your enabling effect whenever you adopt any Immune Booster in this book:

1. Write down your goal. That might be to drop your body mass index from 30 to 25.

2. Divide your goal into a series of easy-to-attain mini-goals.

3. The elation of achieving your first mini-goal then empowers you to achieve your second mini-goal. As success breeds success, your enabling effect propels you on to reach your third, fourth and fifth mini-goals. And so on.

4. Set mini-goals that are relatively easy to attain. If your target is to drop your BMI from 30 to 25, divide it into 10 easy steps of half a point each. Instead of aiming for 25, aim for 29.5 as your first mini-goal. This is merely one-tenth of your total target drop. IBs #5, #8 and #9 should help you achieve this mini-goal quite easily.

As you achieve this small step, the feedback you experience propels you on toward the next mini-goal, a BMI of 29. By attributing each success to your own efforts, your enabling effect will spur you to reach ever lower levels of BMI.

Each time you see an improvement, it provides powerful confirmation that you indeed have control over your BMI and that you yourself can often do as much or more to beat obesity than any drug or treatment given to you by someone else.

To track your success day by day, you must keep a diary.

Only by keeping careful records can you detect the often slow but discernible drops in BMI. Note the date and time of each measurement. Describe any circumstances that seem related to your progress, such as the levels of stress you experience at home and at work, what you ate and drank, the side effects of any medications and, if you're female, any association with oral contraceptives or menstrual periods. A diary is also an excellent diagnostic tool for your doctor's guidance.

One immunologist estimates that when the enabling and placebo effects function together, they rack up the competence of the immune system by at least 45 percent.

The Endorphin Effect: How It Sparks Immunity and KOs Pain

"Runner's high" is another name for the endorphin effect, a giant pain-killer that lurks in the mind. But you don't have to run to release it. A brisk walk, swim or bicycle ride for 35 minutes should create an incredible feeling of well-being that lifts the spirits, suppresses both pain and depression and stabilizes the emotions for the rest of the day.

Actually, any brisk, rhythmic exercise continued for 35 minutes releases clouds of tiny peptide molecules in the brain called *endorphins*. These natural narcotics switch off pain and depression by binding to pain receptors. As they block the receptors, they wipe out depression and anxiety and boost self-esteem. They also build a strong self-image that lasts until bedtime. Above all, endorphins are powerful boosters of mood and immunity.

A 1995 study by Martha Storandt, Ph.D. (reported in that year's *Journal of Gerontology*) demonstrated the ability of endorphins to reduce pain. Researchers examined 87 healthy people aged 60 to 73 who then participated in a 12-month program of rhythmic exercise and flexibility training.

Dr. Storandt found that exercise not only releases endorphins but significantly boosts our sense of self-confidence, morale, self esteem and well-being. All enhance our immuno-competence. No improvement was found in a control group of 34 people who did not exercise. These results led Dr. Storandt to suggest that exercise for older people should be as routine as brushing your teeth.

To start your endorphins flowing, begin with a low-intensity exercise like walking 3 to 4 times a week for up to 30 minutes. As your fitness improves, work up to walking-swimming-bicycling for 35 minutes at a fairly brisk pace. The pace should be sufficiently fast to speed up your breathing and heart rate and (swimming excepted) cause mild perspiration to appear on the brow in warm weather.

The endorphin effect lasts only until you fall asleep. But you can get it back next morning by exercising again. This is the pain-killing component of our healing-regeneration system. People who suffer from chronic pain usually exercise immediately after they wake up. This way they experience pain relief throughout the day until bedtime.

As you walk, swim or pedal your blues away, compare the powerful feeling of accomplishment that you experience to the feeling of helplessness and passivity that so frequently accompanies dependence on antidepressants or other pharmaceuticals.

The Immune-Rallying Power of the Knowledge
Effect

Several hospital studies have demonstrated that the more a patient knows and understands about her disease and how her treatment functions, the more likely she is to believe it will succeed.

A basic principle of all self-healing is to learn as much as possible about your disorder. The literature is filled with case histories of people who achieved a considerable degree of control over their disease by simply learning all there was to know about it. At least one documented study confirms that you can conquer arthritis pain by simply understanding more about the disease.

When Dr. Kate Lorig of Stanford University studied a group of 224 arthritis patients, she found that educating them about their disorder reduced pain as effectively as any of the current arthritis medications. During the 4-year study, members of the test group who received the education made 43 percent fewer visits to a physician than did members of the control group who received no arthritis instruction.

Researchers have found that knowing how everything works makes it much easier to believe in. And the stronger our belief, the more it turns on the placebo effect.

MAKE YOURSELF A MEDICALLY EDUCATED
LAYPERSON

You can understand and learn more about the immune system by reading this book. Eventually, you may know as much about the immune system as your doctor does. Besides

34

giving your immunity a leg-up, this knowledge helps you make intelligent choices and decisions about which Immune Boosters to use. It also helps you work as a partner with your doctor.

Chapters 2 and 3 provide a clear, scientifically based explanation of the immune system and how it works to beat cancer and infections. Reading about each Immune Booster will then expand your knowledge further.

CHAPTER TWO

Understanding Immunity: How the Immune System Works and Why

One of the best ways to supercharge your immunity is to learn more about it. For starters, we should never underestimate its power.

Though it consists of microscopic cells and molecules visible only through a powerful microscope, the immune system is a belligerant fighting machine totally dedicated to defending the body. In fact, it can become so aggressive that, in certain cases, it can get out of control and begin attacking the body itself.

If it weren't for cells called *T-suppressors* that dampen its fighting urge, the immune system could become so belligerent that armies of immune cells mobilized to repel an invader could rampage through the bloodstream out of control and looking for something else to attack.

This is exactly what happens when a person gets rheumatoid arthritis. This disease is caused when the immune system runs amok and attacks cartilage in body joints. Or it may attack other body organs, causing a litany of diseases ranging from lupus to ankylosing spondylitis, multiple sclerosis, pernicious anemia, scleroderma, Type I (juvenile onset) diabetes or ulcerative colitis. All are known as autoimmune diseases because they are caused by an immune system gone awry.

Another type of immune cell called a *natural killer* lurks in lymph nodes ready to annihilate any cancer cell or any foreign invader that enters the body. In the process of battling the hepatitis B virus, for example, natural killer cells may destroy the entire liver, causing a person to die. Yet this ferocious killer is easily subdued by emotional stress.

Other cells patrol the bloodstream on a constant seek-and-destroy mission, while millions of others await a signal to begin manufacturing missile-like antibodies that can paralyze and kill an invading microbe.

But before most immune cells can attack an invader, they must be given permission by certain key cells called *helpers*. When these helper cells are themselves the target of a virus—as in AIDS—much of the immune system becomes frozen and unable to act.

WHO'S WHO IN THE IMMUNE SYSTEM

Obviously, the immune system is a highly complex and sophisticated organization, unbelievably ferocious when attacking unfriendly viruses or cells, yet itself easily knocked

37

down by negative emotions, a host of health-destroying life-style habits or an immune-deficiency disease such as AIDS.

Nonetheless, we ourselves have the power to keep it super-charged and free of the imbalances that cause autoimmu-nity. Before we can do so, however, we need to learn all we can about this unseen power within.

So the first step in boosting your immune power is to become familiar with each type of immune cell and with some of the terminology that immunologists use. You can then put this knowledge to work to make yourself as disease-proof as it is humanly possible to become.

Let's begin by learning who's who in the immune system and the role that each of the characters play in the overall immune response. (If you encounter a few terms before their meaning has been explained, keep reading. The meaning of almost all names and terms is explained as this chapter unfolds.)

For easier understanding, I have omitted some of the less important immune functions as well as some of the more obscure and difficult-to-pronounce terms.

All white cells in the bloodstream are immune cells, and immunologists call them *leukocytes*. Most leukocytes are born as neophyte cells in the marrow of the body's long bones. As they grow, some neophyte cells migrate to the thymus gland where they mature as T-cells. Others remain in the bone marrow and mature as B-cells.

Collectively, T- and B-cells are known as *lymphocytes*. Immunologists usually refer to them as T-lymphocytes or B-lymphocytes.

The Thymus: The Body's School for T-Cells

A small gray gland located atop the heart, the thymus is the center of the immune system. During their sojourn in the thymus, each student T-cell learns to recognize one of over a million antigens which exist in the human environment. An *antigen* is a molecular recognition code carried on the surface of every cell or virus. It identifies unfriendly microbes as nonself and as a target to be attacked.

Each T-cell is programmed to recognize only a single antigen. For instance, a single T-cell may be programmed to identify a part of an influenza virus. But various T-cells are each specific for just one of the million antigens that humans may encounter.

While in the thymus, T-cells also learn to recognize a set of proteins displayed on the walls of our own body cells which identifies them as self and friendly and not to be attacked. Any T-cell which fails to recognize the self as friendly is killed in the thymus. Yet an occasional one is believed to survive and become capable of triggering an autoimmune disease later on.

Though it's not quite clear how, all leukocytes also learn to recognize bacteria that live and work in the body as friendly and self. Much of our digestion is actually carried out by these bacteria, yet the immune system has somehow learned to leave them alone.

During the first few years of life, the thymus works overtime to educate billions of T-cells. It then begins to atrophy and T-cell production dwindles. Since each T-cell lives for 60 to 65 years, most people are fairly well protected against disease until around age 70. But after that, T-cell function begins to diminish and older people become more susceptible to infections and cancer.

As T-cells mature in the thymus, they adopt one of four different functions. Immunologists call this *differentiation* and label T-cells with the identifying letters CD meaning *cluster of differentiation*. For example, a helper T-cell bears the label CD4, or it may simply be called a *T4-cell*.

39

The Principal Classes of T-Cells

The four principal classes of T-cells include helper, suppessor, killer and natural killer cells.

Helper T-Cells

Helper T-cells (CD4 or T4-cells) are alarm-sounders. When an unfriendly antigen is detected in the bloodstream, they turn on and orchestrate the entire immune response.

Helper T-cells are activated when a macrophage cell (described later) displays a piece of antigen from an invading virus or bacteria. As a T4-cell specific to this antigen recognizes the antigen, it secretes *cytokines*, chemical messengers that authorize other lymphocytes to begin to attack the invading microbe. Without permission from a T4-cell, most other lymphocytes are unable to take part in the immune response or to begin manufacturing antibodies.

Suppressor T-Cells

Suppressor T-cells (CD8 or T8-cells) work in tandem with helper T-cells to regulate and control the intensity of an immune response. As soon as an invader is defeated, they secrete a cytokine that suppresses the immune attack and maintains the immune system in equilibrium until another invader is identified.

Killer T-Cells

Killer T-cells kill by secreting a toxin which they inject into the antigen of a foreign invader through a hollow tube that they project. Before a killer T-cell can attack, it must first receive permission from a helper T-cell. Killer T-cells

40

will attack a body cell if that cell contains a virus. They also attack cancer cells and implanted organs.

Natural Killer Cells

Natural killer (NK) cells are actually primitive T-cells that are free to attack indiscriminately without requiring permission from a helper T-cell. This makes them the immune system's first line of defense. Since they look receptors for identifying antigen, NK cells work best when their target has first been identified by macrophages and helper T-cells. These cells release the chemical messenger interferon (described below) which attracts and stimulates NK cells, causing them to grow larger and more aggressive.

NK cells also zero in readily on targets that have already been coated with antibodies such as tumor cells and body cells infected with a virus. NK cells swiftly migrate through the bloodstream to such targets which they immediately kill with their toxic enzymes.

Cytokines: Communication Lines of the Immune System

It's difficult to realize that these life-and-death struggles take place between organisms so microscopic that one millionth part of a quart of blood contains approximately 850 helper T-cells and 500 NK cells. The total number of T-cells in the body runs into the hundreds of billions. All these T-cells and all other leukocytes communicate with one another by secreting hormonelike chemical messengers called *cytokines*.

Cytokines produced by lymphocytes are also known as

lymphokines. Interferon, another cytokine, is released by T-cells and macrophages. And interleukins are widely used for communication by all leukocytes in just about every immune reaction.

Lymphokines

Lymphokines are used by T-cells to authorize B-cells to begin manufacturing antibodies. Other T-cells secrete lymphokines to lure more T-cells to an infection site.

Interferon

Interferon is released by T-cells and macrophages to guide NK cells to a target site. It is also used to prevent viruses from multiplying inside body cells. Interferon has also slowed the rate of cancer growth in animals (but less so in humans since the human body reacts adversely to large amounts of interferon).

Interleukins: The Immune System's Molecular Triggers

Ten or more different series of interleukins (IL) exist, each carrying a different message to a different group of cells. Only three will be discussed here.

IL-1

IL-1 activates the temperature control center in the brain and speeds up the immune response by causing a fever in the infected area. Fever is frequently used by the immune system to fight a general body infection. For instance, raising the body temperature 1, 2 or 3 degrees is sufficient to help kill large numbers of influenza virus.

IL-1 can also induce sleep and fatigue and break down muscle cells. It can also stimulate T-cells to produce more IL-2.

IL-2

IL-2 is secreted by helper T-cells to authorize killer T-cells to attack an invader, such as a cancer cell, in the immediate vicinity. It also stimulates all T-cells that are specific to an invader's antigen to release more IL-2.

IL-3

IL-3 is released by lymphocytes to speed up production of neophyte cells in bone marrow, especially when more B, T and NK cells are needed.

Perhaps you're wondering how all these millions of messenger chemicals can float around in the bloodstream without getting mixed up. Actually, the immune system does get its signals crossed when too many cytokines are released simultaneously. An excessive number of cytokines affects the central nervous system, creating a variety of conditions from muscle twitching to allergies and chronic fatigue syndrome.

B-Cells and Antibodies

The role of B-cells is to manufacture antibodies. B-cells are relatively short-lived, and new ones are being constantly produced in the marrow of the body's long bones.

While maturing in the bone marrow, each B-cell becomes specific for only one of the million or so antigens in the

43

human environment. As they mature, B-cells take up stations in the body's lymph nodes. Once there, each B-cell displays its specific antigen on a site on its surface.

When activated T4 cells see a B-cell displaying the antigen of an invading microbe, they secrete chemical messengers to authorize that B-cell to produce antibodies.

The B-cell immediately begins to multiply into a huge number of plasma cells. Each plasma cell can produce millions of antibodies. Antibody production may take several days. But once production begins, the antibodies are deployed into the bloodstream. Carried along by the blood flow, they glide throughout the body like missiles, each seeking an antigen it can lock on to and disable.

Antibodies are Y-shaped protein molecules. Using their two upper arms, each antibody locks on to a pair of the invader's antigens like a key fitting into a lock. The invader may be a bacteria, a cancer cell or a virus. When a cluster of antibodies coats an invader's surface, a small pathogen like a virus may be completely crippled. Larger pathogens, including tumor cells, may not be totally disabled. But they are so subdued that they are easily destroyed by other immune cells.

Antibodies are also known as *immunoglobulins*, and they play a key role in defending the body against cancer and infections. You'll understand their function better when you learn that there are four principal classes, each defined by the role they play. The classes are IgA, IgE, IgG and IgM (the letters "Ig" stand for immunoglobulin).

IgA

Found in tears, saliva and on fluids which coat the mucous membranes, these immunoglobulins are our first line of defense against invading viruses and other microbes. IgA immunoglobulins abound on the mucuous membranes which line the mouth, nostrils, intestinal tract, bladder and vagina. Here they immobilize and hold pathogens until they are carried out of the body by mucous fluids.

IgE

These immunoglobulins bind to the surface of large *mast cells* that line the nostrils. Mast cells contain a variety of chemicals, including histamine, that are particularly effective in destroying parasites. When an IgE immunoglobulin encounters its matching antigen, it triggers the mast cell to spill out its chemicals and disable the pathogen. But the histamine is also frequently responsible for setting off an allergic reaction.

IgG

The largest and most common immunoglobulin, IgG cripples microorganisms by coating them with a layer of antibodies. Various subtypes specialize in destroying either sugar-coated or nonsugar-coated bacteria, while others disable viruses that seek safety inside cell walls.

IgM

These are primitive immunoglobulins that circulate in the bloodstream and disable any bacteria they encounter. Their effectiveness is somewhat diminished by their large size which prevents them from penetrating body tissue.

45

How Complement Helps Antibodies Kill Pathogenic Bacteria

Complement is a series of eleven chemicals which act as enzymes or catalysts in antigen-antibody reactions. Whenever an IgG or IgM immunoglobulin binds on to an antigen, this act releases the first chemical. This chemical then triggers the release of the second chemical and so on until all eleven have been released.

Each chemical step produces a different enzyme reaction. One step dilates blood vessels while another destroys the walls of the bacteria. In one step, incompatible red blood cells are destroyed; in another scavenger cells called *phagocytes* are attracted to an infection site. In yet another step, complement helps to neutralize viruses. In each step, complement works closely with antibodies to kill unfriendly microbes.

But one complement step, designed to make blood vessels constrict, has an unfortunate side effect. It triggers mast cells in the nostrils to release histamine in quantities so large that it often results in a severe allergic reaction.

The Immune System Never Forgets

After manufacturing a specific antibody, plasma cells often become memory cells for that antibody. That is, they memorize that one single antigen and they carry it for years or even for life. Should that same antigen enter the body again, it is quickly recognized by memory cells specific to that antigen. Response is swift and the invader is destroyed before the disease has a chance to begin.

As a group, memory cells are able to memorize every antigen which has ever triggered the immune response. In

46

reality, millions of memory cells exist for each of these antigens.

Memory cells make us immune to diseases like measles and mumps after a first initial attack. By exposing lymphocytes to a harmless amount of antigen, vaccination uses the same memory mechanism to immunize us against a score of common infections.

Phagocyte Cells: Giants of the Immune System

Phagocytes are a class of giant scavenger cells that includes macrophages, polys, mast cells and basophils. All are born in the bone marrow and mature swiftly. Some, like macrophages, then patrol the bloodstream, while others lie in wait for an invader in the liver or spleen.

Macrophages

Besides engulfing microbes killed by other leukocytes, these large scavenger cells play a variety of roles. Using their pseudopods, or tentacle-like arms, macrophages can entrap invading microbes and chop their surface into small segments containing sample antigens.

Certain macrophages called *antigen presenting cells* (APCs) display one of these antigen samples on their outer surface. Passing T4-cells then review this sample. When a helper T-cell arrives that is specific for this sample antigen, that cell is activated. Almost immediately, the T4-cell triggers the immune response, and all cells are alerted to attack any microbe bearing this same antigen.

Macrophages also process invading microbes for easy recognition by other lymphocytes and antibodies.

47

Polymorphonuclear Cells

Also called *polys* (or granulocytes or neutrophils), these large cells have several lobes and can transform themselves into a variety of shapes. Polys specialize in destroying bacteria. They are lured to the site of an invader by chemicals released by the complement system.

Once a poly detects this chemical, it speeds through the bloodstream toward the pathogen and kills it by releasing granules of toxic enzymes called *lysosomes*. One variety of poly can release lysosomes powerful enough to break through the walls of an invading parasite.

Inflammation: Another Weapon to Fight Infection

Phagocytes, particularly mast cells and basophils, release chemical enzymes to draw other lymphocytes to an infection site. Called mediators, these chemicals consist of histamine, leukotrienes and prostaglandins. As they are released, they cause reddening, swelling and tenderness which we know as inflammation. Inflammation is a protective mechanism used by the immune system to help kill foreign invaders. It is also a prominent symptom of several autoimmune diseases, particularly rheumatoid arthritis.

Complement and interferon are also involved in provoking inflammation as are other substances secreted by specialized T4-cells. The inflammation process is regulated by prostaglandins (hormone-like molecules involved in almost every body function). Aspirin reduces inflammation by blocking production of the type of prostaglandin which turns on the inflammation process.

Bacteria: Unwelcome Invaders that Poison the Body

While billions of friendly bacteria live in our intestines and aid in digestion, the unfriendly types that invade the body are a form of plant cell that cause illness and damage. Once in the body, most bacteria are recognized as nonself and the immune system swiftly strikes back.

Antibodies are the immune system's first line of defense against a bacterial invasion. By locking on to receptors on bacteria cells, antibodies paralyze and disable these cells and prevent them from releasing their toxins. As the cells die, they release immune-complex, a mixture of chemicals from antibodies and bacteria that frequently triggers inflammation and fever.

Among common bacterial infections are botulism, which attacks the nervous system, cholera, diphtheria, tetanus, tuberculosis and whooping cough, which frequently hits young children and older people. Even a vigorous immune system is not able to successfully fight off all bacterial invasions. Were it not for antibiotics, the death rate from bacterial diseases would be much higher than it is today.

Viruses: Fast-Acting Foes of Immunity

As the most common and frequent invaders of the body, viruses are the primary targets of immune system attack. A virus is simply a piece of DNA or similar genetic material encapsulated in a coating of protein or fat. It is so incredibly microscopic that 5 billion viruses can exist in a single drop of blood.

Although they are a near-life form, viruses are not alive.

49

They can reproduce only by entering a living cell. Once inside a body cell, their protective coating melts away, freeing their genetic material to hijack the cell.

Immediately, the virus's genetic material orders the host cell to become a virus factory. Thousands of copies of the virus are manufactured. So many are produced that the cell bursts and disgorges a horde of new viruses into the bloodstream. The new viruses are then carried into other cells, and the process is repeated ad infinitum.

Since they are not alive, viruses are simply carried about by air and water currents, by people and animals and by the bloodstream. Most are passed from one person to another by inhaling air-borne particles, kissing, sexual contact or touching the nose and mouth with the fingers. They enter the body through a body opening or through a bite, cut, or needle prick.

Once in the bloodstream, they bond with receptors on the surface of a cell for which they are specific. Many viruses carry receptors that are specific for only a single type of cell. Hepatitis B viruses may bond only with liver cells. Once on the surface of a cell, they are swept inside as the cell absorbs nutrients.

Many viruses are life-threatening. Others, such as the hundred or so different rhinoviruses that cause the common cold, are self-limiting. They are wiped out by the immune system in a matter of days. Others, like Hepatitis B, are able to enter and infect millions of cells in the liver. Each of these infected cells must be destroyed by NK and killer T-cells aided by complement, interferon and billions of antibodies. In severe cases, the immune system must wipe out every cell in the liver, causing the death of the host.

Viruses Outwit Immunity with Antigenic Drift

Viruses have developed sophisticated methods to escape detection. Over time, viruses are able to change their antigens in a process called *antigenic drift*. Influenza virus is subject to antigenic drift each year. Each summer, public health officials make an educated guess as to the actual antigen which the influenza virus may adopt the following winter. Influenza vaccine is then manufactured specifically for this antigen. Occasionally, the officials are wrong, and the body is left unprotected with no memory cells that carry the invader's antigen.

Retroviruses ("retro" means to turn around) have a special form of genetic material called RNA (ribo nucleic acid). These viruses escape detection by releasing an enzyme which transforms their RNA into a slightly different form of genetic material called DNA.

HIV is a well-known form of retrovirus. It carries receptors specific for human helper T-cells. As the HIV virus multiplies out of control inside helper T-cells, it disorients the entire immune response, setting the stage for AIDS.

Currently, few medications, including antibiotics, are effective against viruses. The best protection is a combination of vaccinations, a supercharged immune system and the protective techniques described in the various Immune Boosters in this book.

THE ANATOMY OF AN IMMUNE RESPONSE

The following is an updated version of the immune system's response to an invasion by cold viruses, taken from my

51

earlier book *Eighteen Natural Ways to Beat the Common Cold.*

It was a Friday afternoon in mid-February and Bob Rhinehart, a 35-year-old Florida real estate salesman, was on his way to a closing party. The gathering was to honor Jack Fetterman, another salesman who had just closed an important deal.

Bob greeted Jack with a hearty handshake.

"How's it feel to make five grand in a day?" Bob asked, as he picked up a chicken drumstick and began gnawing.

"Oh, the money's great, of course," Jack answered. "But I think I'm coming down with something. My nose feels dry and tight. There's a scratchy sensation in my throat. And somehow I don't feel quite up to par."

Jack's surmise proved correct. He spent the weekend at home, nursing one of the most virulent colds he'd ever experienced. To avoid giving his cold to others, Jack also stayed home on Monday. But despite Jack's good intentions, it was already too late. The common cold becomes contagious almost a day before any symptoms appear.

Moments before Jack and Bob shook hands, Jack had touched his nose. When he shook hands with Bob, 10 million microscopic cold viruses were transferred to Bob's hand. A moment later, Bob touched his face as he gnawed on the drumstick. This move placed at least 8 million viruses at the entrance to his nostrils.

As 5 million viral invaders burst into his nose, Bob's body became a battleground for an invisible yet incredibly complex war between his immune system and the legions of invading viruses.

Almost two weeks were to pass before Bob's defenses were able to rout the penetrating microorganisms and emerge victorious. It was this desperate life-and-death battle within his own body that created all of Bob's distressing cold symptoms:

the perpetually runny nose, the endless sniffles, the bouts of sneezing, the raw, burned skin around the nostrils and, later in the week, the sore throat and loss of his voice.

Microbial Armies Invade Bob's Nostrils

Within minutes of arriving, most of the viruses were inhaled into Bob's nostrils. Many were immediately trapped like flies on flypaper by the wet, sticky mucosa lining his nasal passages. Legions of cilia—whiplike hairs beating continually in unison at 600 sweeps per minute—then pushed these trapped invaders steadily toward Bob's gullet and down his digestive tract to be destroyed by stomach acids.

But about half the invaders managed to evade the beating cilia. They binded with receptors on some of the millions of body cells lining Bob's nasal passages.

As soon as Bob's nasal cells sensed the presence of a hostile invader, they signaled for help. They released microscopic amounts of a hormone-like chemical messenger in the bloodstream that alerted the immune system. Swiftly, all nearby macrophages and helper T-cells headed for the infection site.

A rhinovirus is the type of virus most frequently responsible for causing the common cold. Consisting of a mere 600 atoms—so small they can be seen only under an electron microscope—the rhinovirus is shaped like a geodesic dome, composed of 20 triangular-shaped facets.

A cunning strategy developed by rhinoviruses has been to place their antigens in a deep, hard-to-reach cleft in each of their facets. These subterfuges allow the rhinovirus to trick its way past the vigilantes of the immune system—the giant macrophage cells.

As the viruses fanned out through Bob's nasal passages,

53

each macrophage within range closed in on a virus. Then, using their arm-like pseudopods, the macrophages groped deep within the clefts on the viruses' surfaces. Some were able to pluck out a viral antigen.

With their pseudopods, the macrophages chopped the antigens into smaller units. Then each macrophage displayed a piece of the virus's antigen side by side with a piece of its own antigen, identifying them as self and friendly. This lessened the risk that an overzealous lymphocyte would mistakenly attack Bob's own cells.

Helper T-Cells Unleash the Immune Response

Each passing helper T-cell then briefly reviewed the antigen samples. But soon, perhaps within seconds, one or more T4-cells arrived, each specific to the viral antigen. The mere act of reading the viral antigen activated the helper T-cells.

Upon becoming activated, each helper T-cell released a variety of lymphokines that alerted every component in Bob's immune system and identified the target. All killer T-cells in the area were authorized to attack the invaders. As each killer T-cell prepared to attack, it released interferon, which interferes with the ability of viruses to multiply.

Meanwhile, the activated T4-cells lost no time in proliferating until millions of lymphocytes had been produced. As they appeared, these new T-cells differentiated into helpers, suppressors and killers. Each recognized the same antigen and all joined in the attack on the viruses.

Throughout his body, each of Bob's cells displayed a set of proteins on its surface that revealed the cell's contents. Each body cell sheltering a virus displayed a sample of the virus. In this way, helper T-cells could recognize each virus-infected cell and mark it for destruction.

54

While this was going on, other helper T-cells raced to Bob's lymph nodes. There they released lymphokine messengers to alert B-cells specific for the virus's antigen. The lymphokines authorized the B-cells to begin producing antibodies. Right away, each B-cell began to multiply into a vast number of plasma cells. And each plasma cell began to manufacture millions of antibodies.

This constant interchange of cytokines between Bob's immune components orchestrated and amplified the attack. Virtually every immune component interacted with and supported all the other components.

Health-Destroying Habits Inhibit Bob's Immune Response

But such a massive build-up is possible only when immuno-competence is high. The ability of our immune system to destroy invaders is a reflection of our own physical and mental health. When we exercise regularly, eat lots of fruits and vegetables and have a positive, upbeat and hopeful attitude, our immuno-competence is enhanced.

Had Bob's lifestyle been built around such factors, his immune system might have conquered the cold in a few brief days. Unfortunately, Bob had been recently divorced. He seldom exercised any more. He lived largely on hamburgers, coffee and fast foods. And he often experienced bouts of lingering depression. As a result, his immuno-competence was so suppressed that his cold lingered on for 12 misery-filled days before his immune system could finally erase it.

Regardless of the competence of one's immune system, the same step-by-step conflict occurs as in Bob's case. The only difference is the speed at which the immune system responds and fights back. A person with a supercharged immunity may be able to throw off a cold as early as the end of the second day.

Yet no matter how high one's immuno-competence, in the beginning the immune system is largely unprepared and helpless to stop the tidal wave of besieging viruses. Millions of rhinoviruses were immediately able to bind on to receptors on cells in the walls of Bob's nose.

In response to the pressure on its surface, each cell puckered up around the virus—and possibly believing it to be a nutrient—innocently absorbed the microorganism into its interior. In the process, each host cell released an enzyme that removed the virus's protein coat. This left the virus core exposed—a tiny piece of translucent RNA containing its genetic code for reproduction.

Once a virus enters a cell in this way, it shuts down the cell's own genetic software and the virus's genetic software takes over. In response to this new programming, Bob's cells each turned out between 100 and 1,000 clones of the virus's genetic package. Included in the viral genes were instructions for the cell to reencapsulate each new virus core in a protein coat.

Day One: Germ Warfare Within

Twenty-four hours after the viruses first arrived, Bob was still unaware of the lonely battle being fought in his body. He had no cold symptoms and still felt fine.

But by now at least a million cells in his nasal passages had been commandeered and transformed into virus factories. Some cells already contained a thousand copies of the original virus invader. Each commandeered cell displayed a tell-tale sample virus on its outer surface, alerting immune cells to the viruses within.

Teaming up, NK and killer T-cells attacked the hemor-rhaging nasal cells, spraying the viruses with paralyzing tox-ins. But as each cell burst open, releasing up to a thousand more viruses, the lymphocytes were overwhelmed. Floating along on the breath, nearly a billion new viruses began to migrate all over Bob's upper-respiratory passages, penetrating his sinuses and the Eustachian tubes that led to his ears and working down to his tonsils, adenoids and throat. Mean-while, infected cells that had hemorrhaged began dying in droves. To prevent blood loss, the immune system sent fi-brinogen, a clotting agent, to dry up the blood in Bob's nasal membranes.

At this point, still without any cold symptoms, Bob be-came contagious. As had happened with his friend Jack the day before, should Bob touch his nose and then touch some-one else's hand or face, the probability was high that he would transmit some of his own rhinoviruses to that person.

Although Bob wasn't coughing or sneezing, he expelled millions of viruses into the air with a strong exhalation. Trav-eling on invisible molecules of water vapor floating in the air, these viruses were then inhaled by other people. While the majority of colds are transmitted by hand-to-hand con-tact, or by touching an object recently handled by a cold victim, colds may also be caught by inhaling air in a room occupied by someone infected with a cold virus. What com-plicates the task of preventing colds is that someone can be contagious while still free of all cold symptoms.

Day Two: The Body Fights Back

At this point, virus production had far outstripped the manufacture of lymphocytes by Bob's immune system. For every virus destroyed by lymphocytes, a hundred thousand

57

more were ready to replace it. By now, however, some of Bob's B-cells had commenced antibody manufacture. Dwelling unseen in the lymph nodes and spleen, B-cells are able to produce thousands of antibodies in a single minute. But in a person with poor immuno-competence, gearing up for this kind of production *can* take several days. Once in production, however, antibodies can lock on to the viruses' antigens, hampering their travel, making them functionally impotent and marking them as targets for destruction by phagocytes.

As T4-cells sized up the invader, they authorized Bob's B-cells to manufacture more than one type of antibody. In this way, several different types of antibodies can each lock on to a different type of receptor on the invading pathogen. Usually, T4-cells instruct plasma cells to produce antibodies in the order most likely to be needed.

At first, Bob's plasma cells turned out only IgM immunoglobulins. Intended only for temporary use against his present cold, they faded away a few days after the cold was overcome. Later, some of Bob's plasma cells were instructed to produce IgG immunoglobulins, a more permanent antibody that would live for several years or even for a lifetime. Should this same virus ever invade Bob's nasal passages again, these antibodies would be instantly available to stop the infection on the spot.

Although reinforcements of NK and killer T-cells were by now hastening to Bob's nose, the viral enemy was still so enormous that only antibodies could finish them off.

Forty-eight hours after the first viruses arrived, at least half the healthy cells in Bob's nasal passages had been infected. As millions of dead and dying cells accumulated in his nose, nasal mast cells began to secrete histamine, which boosts blood flow to the nose and causes inflammation and congestion. In turn, this stimulates membranes to produce copious amounts of mucous to wash away the dead viruses and cells. Inflammation is, therefore, a natural defense mechanism which plays an essential role in the immune response.

As these changes gradually occurred, Bob became vaguely aware of an oncoming cold. He felt a mild but scratchy tickling sensation in his throat. His nose and throat seemed dry. He lost his usual hearty appetite and felt mildly fatigued. And as the day wore on, it became increasingly apparent that a bad cold was approaching. By evening, both his nostrils were completely blocked as mucous flowed like water. Bob experienced bouts of uncontrollable sneezing. His eyes began to water and he had a mild headache. His neck felt swollen and his throat felt sore. He felt tired, feverish and completely miserable.

Day Three: Cold Symptoms Are Healing Processes at Work

After a fitful night, Bob woke feeling thoroughly uncomfortable. As did hundreds of others in his city that day, Bob called in sick, took two aspirin, drank plenty of fluids and stayed in bed.

What Bob and most others failed to realize is that cold symptoms, uncomfortable as they seem, are a clear indication that the immune system is taking strong defensive measures.

What we call a cold is really the symptoms of the healing process. The swelling and tenderness in Bob's neck, and his sore throat were direct proof that a vigorous immune response was under way in the lymph nodes in his neck. (Lymph nodes are narrow, pea-sized vessels in the lymph system where lymphocytes live and battle with invaders.) Other lymph glands exist under the arms and in the groin. These, too, may become tender and swollen, as lymphocyte populations mushroom during an immune response.

Bob's ceaselessly runny nose was also part of his immune system's defense against further viral invasion. And the inflammation in his nasal passages was part of his immune response to contain the spread of infection. Unfortunately, the swollen tissue and free-flowing fluids exerted pressure on nerve endings, causing unceasing misery and discomfort.

While fever isn't generally associated with colds, the immune system frequently employs fever in its battle with influenza and other viruses that invade the body's respiratory tract. Most of these viruses have been living for thousands of years in human air passages at a temperature slightly below that of our normal core temperature of 98.6°F. These viruses are extremely sensitive to temperature change. In its efforts to destroy these invaders, the immune system may raise the core temperature to as high as 104°.

This rise of several degrees is enough to immobilize billions of influenza and other viruses as well as other pathological organisms. Fever, then, is a natural immune response to get rid of invading viruses. You can shorten the duration of many infections by allowing the body to maintain its fever and avoiding the use of any medication or aspirin to lower your temperature. Unless your temperature is really excessive (104° or higher), a fever is a sign that your body is basically healthy and is fighting the infection. (Caution: Temperatures of 104° or more usually warrant immediate medical attention.)

Although the common cold can lead to complications, by itself it's almost never fatal. Eventually, even the weakest among us muster sufficient antibodies to ensure its demise. Techni-

60

cally, the common cold is considered a self-limiting, upper-respiratory-tract infection, and in most people, the immune system can annihilate it in under fourteen days.

However, in people with supercharged immunity, a cold is often stopped dead in its tracks by the end of the second or third day after symptoms first appear.

Day Four: Poor Immunity Delays Bob's Recovery

Although some of the cold medications Bob took dulled his discomfort, none affected the course of his cold. As the fourth day dawned, billions of plasma cells toiled within Bob's body to speed up antibody production. But his mediocre level of immuno-competence hampered their efforts. As a result, his immune system took eight days to accomplish what a person with stronger immunity might have achieved in 36 hours.

On this day, Bob managed to drag himself out of bed. Despite the misery he was enduring, he forced himself to go to work.

His constantly stuffed-up nose caused Bob to breathe through his mouth. No longer was the air he inhaled cleansed, warmed and moistened by his nasal cilia and mucous membranes. An endless postnasal drip also irritated his throat.

Days Five to Fourteen: Bob's Immune System
Finally Triumphs

A week after the viruses first entered his nose, they were able to infect the vocal cords in Bob's throat. His voice became a mere croak and he was constantly hoarse. However, in his upper air passages, viral production began to taper off, due in part to a shortage of remaining cells to infect.

By the eighth day, while Bob's immune system still struggled with antibody production, he became almost voiceless and his larynx felt swollen and tender to the touch. Bob felt even more depressed than usual and he was unable to relax.

On the ninth day, Bob's compromised immune system finally managed to produce the required antibodies. Sweeping through his lymph and bloodstream, vast populations of antibodies poured on to the viral hordes still occupying his nasal passages. Locking on to antigen receptors on each of the billions of viruses, the IgM and IgG immunoglobulins began to activate a series of complement enzymes.

Together, the antibodies and complement subdued the viruses. They also served as markers for millions of phagocyte cells which literally swallowed the viruses and digested them.

By the tenth day, the full impact of Bob's immune response was unleashed on the viral invaders. Antibodies, complement, NK and killer T-cells and macrophages all attacked the viruses in unison.

Like other immune system components, complement production had been slowed by Bob's poor diet and his other counterproductive lifestyle habits. Defects in his complement system contributed significantly to his susceptibility to laryngitis.

It took several more days for Bob's head cold to disappear and his voiceless and sore throat to clear up. In fact, it was not until the fourteenth day after the initial infection that Bob's immune system had completely vanquished the last of the viruses in his larynx and throat.

Putting the Brakes on the Immune Response

Now that the viruses were gone, Bob's bloodstream was filled with rampaging armies of NK and killer T-cells, macrophages and antibodies all on the lookout for trouble. Thirsting for blood and almost out of control, these aggressive immune system components can mass in joints such as the elbow or knee and, once there, attack the body's own cells in a phenomenon known as *autoimmunity.*

To prevent such a possibility, whenever a target pathogen has been destroyed, suppressor T-cells (T8-cells) act to inhibit the immune response. Sending commands by lymphokines, they turned off all antibody production in Bob's B-cells and halted further attacks by killer cells. Under their urging, Bob's entire immune system gradually slowed to noncombatant status.

Only phagocytes were permitted to continue cruising the blood vessels in his air passages to mop up debris. Within a few days, most of the lymphocytes and antibodies replicated for the conflict had died off. But some lymphocytes would live on in Bob's bloodstream for longer periods. Memory cells would remain sensitive to the specific virus which had produced Bob's cold. For as long as these lympocytes lived, Bob would be immmune to that specific rhinovirus.

As we experience cold after cold during a lifetime—and various strains of influenza and other viral infections—we gradually acquire immunity to an increasing number (though not all). This phenomenon explains why children aged up to 10 or more often catch one cold after another. During these early years, the body is exposed to a continual series of new viruses to which no prior immunity has been developed.

63

Our Immune Power Declines with Advancing Years

Gradually, as we grow older, we acquire immunity to a growing number of cold and other viruses. As a result, colds and certain other infectious diseases become less common with increasing age. But in older people, this advantage is frequently offset by weakening of the entire immune system as we age.

With advancing years, the thymus gland all but disappears. T-cell response then gradually declines, and this, in turn, weakens the response of B-cells and antibodies. As we grow older, the immune system also produces more of the cytokines that trigger inflammation.

But free radical damage is the principal culprit that causes the immune system to lose vigor as we age. (Free radicals are oxidized molecules of dietary fat that create serious damage to the DNA of body cells.) Most immune system cells contain a high level of polyunsaturated fat in their membranes, making them highly susceptible to oxidation by free radicals.

Besides cigarette smoking, the principal promoter of free radicals are fats in the Standard American Diet (SAD). By age 70, the immune system of the average sedentary person eating the Standard American Diet has lost 60 to 70 percent of the competence it had at age 15. IBs #3 and #4 describe how to minimize free radical damage and maintain a high level of immunity for many years longer than the average person of the same age.

Due perhaps to their greater hormone activity, women tend to have stronger and more active immune systems than men. Women also have a stronger antibody response than men, and they have a higher resistance to viral and bacterial infections. But this ability can also backfire, causing women

64

to manufacture more antibodies that attack their own tissue. This explains why women are three times more prone than men to develop most autoimmune diseases. Rheumatoid arthritis, lupus and myasthenia gravis (a muscular dysfunction) strike women three times as often as men.

Although no vaccination yet exists against autoimmune diseases or the common cold, whether you're male or female, one of the best ways throughout life to prevent many of the most common infections is to keep your inoculations up to date.

The Immune System Usually Responds in Much the Same Way

Though fighting a relatively mild virus, the immune response just described is essentially the same reaction that the immune system would make against a more virulent virus, a bacteria, a cancer cell, a fungi or an organ implanted from another person.

In Chapters 5, 6 and 7, the text under each Immune Booster explains more about the way in which the immune system is affected by stress and depression; being overweight or sleep-deprived, by solar exposure, or by exercise, food and nutritional supplements. To expand your knowledge on these topics, look up:

Allergies: IB #14
Diet: IBs #3, #4, #5 and #6
Exercise: IBs #8 and #9
Nutritional supplements and herbs: IBs #1 and #2
Overweight: IBs #3, #4. #5, #6, #8 and #9
Sleep deprivation: IB #13

Solar exposure: IB #12
Stress and depression: IBs #8, #15, #16, #17 and #18

How Physicians Evaluate Your Immunity

The ratio between T-helper and T-suppressor cells helps physicians diagnose disease. One common test is the Cellular Immunity Assay which reveals abnormalities in the immune system by calculating the percentages of various immune system components in the bloodstream and the ratios between them. In a healthy person, the ratio is 1.8 helpers to 1 suppressor. In a person with lupus, the ratio is 1.5 to 1. A lower ratio could indicate HIV or other immune-deficiency disease.

Another test is available to determine autoantibodies, each of which is linked to an autoimmune disease. The level of antibodies such as IgA are also easily measured and give a quick approximation of the overall effectiveness of your immune system. Other tests are available for cancer and rheumatoid arthritis. It may be possible soon to evaluate your immuno-competence with a simple home test kit.

The levels of lymphocytes and phagocytes are also indicated in the standard blood chemistry profile frequently ordered by physicians as part of a medical checkup. While readings may be reduced by an allergy, infection or malignant tumor, they do present a picture of your current immuno-competence.

The Healing Power of Knowledge

If by now you're wondering how on earth you're going to remember each of the many complicated steps in the immune response, relax! Provided you have read through this chapter and have at least absorbed the general idea and some of the terminology, that may be all you need to know. For most of us, it's the effort we make to learn and understand that really counts. If you're like most of us, that's more than enough to turn on your knowledge effect and boost the power of your healing-regeneration system by at least 20 percent.

Chapter 3 then adds to your knowledge by explaining exactly how a body cell becomes cancerous and how the immune system recognizes and annihilates it. Chapter 3 also describes several natural ways to prevent or retard cancer.

How to Stop Cancer Up Front: Before It Overloads the Immune System

E very day it is estimated that between 500 and 10,000 cells become cancerous in the average American's body. The task of finding and destroying each of these cells can overload and weaken a person's immune system. Were our body to suddenly cut cancer cell production by 90 percent, chances are good that our immune system would immediately become supercharged.

This is exactly what can happen if we're willing to prevent the formation of most cancer cells in the first place. This relieves our immune systems of the huge burden of destroying hundreds or thousands of potential tumor cells each day.

I can tell you right now that if you're willing to do what it takes to succeed, you clearly and definitely *can* make yourself almost cancer-proof. It won't happen overnight. But in a few weeks, you could be well on the way.

Are you ready? Then the first step is to understand exactly what cancer is and how it develops.

WHAT EXACTLY IS CANCER?

Cancer is a dysfunction of the genetic blueprint (DNA) in a body cell that causes the cell to begin to multiply rapidly and grow into a tumor.

During a person's lifetime, most normal body cells are programmed to divide and replicate up to a maximum of about 50 times. After that, the cell dies. Normal cells have a limited mortality. But when a cell becomes cancerous, it also becomes immortal. A cancer cell multiplies rapidly. Provided nutrients are available, it continues to divide and grow into a massive tumor containing trillions of cells.

With a few exceptions, every human cell has the potential to become malignant. The process occurs in two steps.

Step One: Cancer Initiation

Each of us is composed of some 60 trillion body cells. At the core of each of these cells is the DNA (deoxyribo nucleic acid), a long double-helix strand containing about 3 billion biochemical characters (genes) that encode the blueprint for a human being.

At each cell division during a person's life, an error may occur in replicating some of the genes strung out along the DNA strands. In a healthy person, proteins slide along the

69

DNA strands, fixing any errors (mutations) that occur during cell division. These repair molecules are often likened to the biological equivalent of a computer spell check. But, occasionally, they miss a mutation. When several mutations are overlooked, a cell may take the first step toward cancer. It is then said to be *initiated.*

Most cells are initiated by a carcinogen such as cigarette smoke, certain hormones or free radicals. Cancer can also be initiated by other carcinogens such as aflatoxin found in mouldy peanuts, asbestos, benzene, chlorine-based prescription drugs, herbicides, radiation, radon or solvents.

The Chemical "Bad Guys" That Explode in Our Cells

But many cancers are diet-related. Free radicals, for instance, are chemical "bad guys" formed when fat consumed in the diet enters the body and reacts with oxygen to form molecules containing unpaired electrons. Once in our cells, these unstable molecules set off a chain reaction. The havoc they create extends to actual physical damage to the genes in our cells.

Intriguing proof came in 1993 when researchers at the University of Washington, Seattle, compared tissue removed from the breasts of healthy women with tissue from cancerous breasts. In every case, tissue from cancerous breasts showed much more oxidation damage caused by free radicals.

But the Standard American Diet contains other carcinogens. Any food that is salt-cured, smoked or pickled — including most sausage and luncheon meats — frequently contains nitrosamines, a potent carcinogen.

70

Yet the tar and nicotine in cigarettes is the single most powerful promoter of free radicals. Even inhaling second-hand smoke can lead to cancer. Women who are heavy smokers have a high risk of developing cervical cancer. And 80 percent of lung cancer is attributable to smoking. By comparison, relatively few cases of cancer are initiated by a defective gene.

One way or another, a body cell becomes initiated with a small number of *oncogenes* (cancer-prone genes in DNA). But the number is insufficient to change the cell's genetic blueprint. Although the cell has been initiated, it is still benign, its molecular structure remains intact and the immune system continues to recognize the cell as friendly and self.

Step Two: Cancer Activation

By middle age, the average American has accumulated several million initiated cells. In a person who exercises regularly, eats plenty of foods that grow on plants and does not smoke, consume alcohol or suffer from stress, relatively few initiated cells ever become cancerous.

The reason is that tumor-suppressor genes in the DNA of every cell stop cell division if it becomes too rapid. In fact, a recently discovered series of multiple-tumor-suppressor genes inhibit tumor formation by preventing cells from dividing abnormally fast.

But even these powerful suppressor genes can fail to work when a cell is bombarded with certain hormones, environmental carcinogens or free radicals. When these toxic chemicals bind to DNA molecules inside a cell, they may cause mutations that accelerate the speed at which a cell divides.

71

In fact, tumor-suppressor genes themselves may be damaged or turned off by environmental carcinogens, free radicals or hormones. Defects in tumor-suppressor genes have been found in half of all cancer cases. When multiple-suppressor genes stop functioning, the result is often a brain tumor, breast or lung cancer or melanoma.

When Is a Cell Activated?

An initiated cell becomes *activated* when carcinogens, free radicals or hormones cause further mutations in several genes at the same time. Other molecular assaults also knock out key tumor-suppressor genes in the initiated cell's genetic code.

Then oncogenes release a telomere-boosting enzyme (telomerase). (The tail end of each strand of DNA is called a *telomere*. Each time a healthy cell divides, the telomeres fray or break off and become shorter. Eventually, after a cell divides about 50 times, telomere loss is so great that the cell ceases to divide and dies.) But telomerase repairs telomere damage. The cell becomes immortal and is then able to divide rapidly. It quickly multiplies into a life-threatening tumor.

When telomere repair so alters a cell's genetic structure that it is no longer recognized as self by the body's leukocytes, it becomes a full-fledged cancer cell. As this occurs, most cells display on their surface the cause of their cancer such as a fragment of a carcinogen. This marker is swiftly recognized as a nonself antigen by patrolling macrophages. Cytokines are released and NK cells move in for the kill.

Some Cancer Markers Are Fuzzy

But not all cancer cells are able to display this tell-tale marker. Other cancer cells may be oddly shaped, or their marker may be incomplete or indistinct. As a result, they may go unrecognized for much longer than, say, the easily recognized antigen of an invading bacteria or virus.

In any case, the immune reaction mounted against a cancer cell is usually less vigorous than that mobilized against an invading microbe. For example, fewer NK cells are alerted than when the body is invaded by foreign microbes.

Particularly if the immune system is weakened by emotional stress or by fighting other pathogens, an activated cell is able to survive. However, once its antigen is clearly recognized, a strong immune response occurs. T4-cells authorize killer T-cells to act and B-cells to manufacture antibodies. Eventually, as antibodies zero in, they cover the cancer cell and subdue it. NK and killer T-cells then finish it off, leaving giant phagocyte cells to pick up the debris.

Activated cells are many times more numerous in people who smoke, are overweight, eat a high-fat diet low in fruits and vegetables, suffer from stress or fail to exercise. That's because each of these factors is a suppressor of immunity or a promoter of free radicals or both. By ceasing to smoke, cutting down on fat, eating many more fruits and vegetables, changing our response to stress and beginning to exercise, we can dramatically reduce the number of cells that are activated in our bodies each day.

We can't change the number of cells that are already initiated. But we can stop initiating more. And we can stop activating those that are already initiated. The way to do it is to read IBs #3, #4, #6 and #8. Adopt these Immune Boosters into your lifestyle and you can slash your risk of ever getting cancer by 50 to 75 percent or possibly more.

73

Can the Immune System Cause a Spontaneous
Remission from Cancer?

On rare occasions, a medically diagnosed cancerous tumor has gone into remission and disappeared without medical treatment, or in spite of it. These cases, it was found, usually follow a life event that prompts a powerful immune response.

Events that seem to lead to a remission have included a biopsy, a severe viral or bacterial infection or a vaccination using killed bacteria. Some investigators believe that remission has been due to a sudden, powerful jump in immunocompetence. Others feel that the body's healing-regeneration system is involved. But no one so far has been able to deliberately promote a spontaneous remission of cancer.

However, most researchers agree that a strong immune response releases potent tumor-destroying molecules called the Tumor Necrosis Factor. Actually a cytokine or messenger molecule, the Tumor Necrosis Factor appears to act as a catalyst to direct the healing-regeneration system to focus on the tumor site.

The pioneering work of Dr. Carl Simonton, a radiation oncologist, and psychotherapist Stephanie Matthews-Simonton, plus that of Herbert Benson, M.D. of Harvard Medical School, suggests that a whole-person approach focusing on visualization may help promote an immune response when the immune system fails to recognize cancer cells as foreign.

Immune-arousing visualization techniques are described in IB #17 while other Immune Booster techniques such as IBs #8, #15, #16 and #18 may also help stimulate an immune response. The Simontons' methods are described in their book *Getting Well Again* (J.P. Tarcher, 1978) and are echoed in Dr. Benson's books on the power of belief.

74

The immune response to cancer cells is often poor because, since cancer cells are our own body cells, the immune system fails to recognize them as foreign. As a result, T4-cells fail to turn on the immune response for a cancer cell. Only NK cells can then attack it, and they may not recognize the antigen.

Actually, just about all T-cells and macrophages can be stimulated to attack cancer cells. Sometimes this occurs during an invasion of bacteria. Researchers at Memorial Sloan Kettering Cancer Center in New York recently discovered that transferring tumor-related cells from one species to another (from a human to a mouse) may also trigger a strong immune system attack against cancer.

At this time, however, the visualization method just mentioned seems to be the best hope for precipitating a spontaneous remission. It is not a substitute for needed medical treatment.

Without a Blood Supply, a Tumor Cannot Grow

Nowadays, an increasing number of investigators believe that spontaneous remission can occur only by blocking angiogenesis. They are focusing on one simple fact: that without a blood supply, a tumor cannot grow. Either it lies dormant or it withers and dies.

Once a malignant tumor begins to grow, its cells divide rapidly until a mass of about 1 million cells has formed. A tumor this size—called a *carcinoma in situ*—is little larger than a BB pellet. Without blood vessels, cells in the center of a carcinoma are cut off from the oxygen and nutrients they need to continue growing.

Tumor cells overcome this problem by secreting Angiogenesis Growth Factor, a substance that coaxes nearby blood

75

vessels to sprout capillaries to supply blood to the tumor. This process is known as *angiogenesis*.

How Metastasis Sends Potential Time Bombs All Over the Body

Once angiogenesis occurs, a tumor can continue to multiply at a wild and rapid pace that is both aggressive and threatening. At the same time, breakaway cells from the tumor can travel through the capilleries to distant parts of the body. And once established there, a cancer cell can multiply into another carcinoma. This process is known as *metastasis*.

Cancer cells that spread through metastasis can survive, even after the original tumor has been surgically removed. Often, a metastasized cancer cell may grow into a tumor at a new site but fail to provoke angiogenesis. Without a blood supply, the tiny tumor lies dormant. And since macrophages and T4-cells travel only through the bloodstream, a dormant tumor can remain undetected by the immune system.

Years may go by before the tumor is able to become angiogenic. Then, typically, a decade or more after the original tumor was surgically removed, the same cancer recurs in a new location.

Currently, tiny tumors of a million cells each are very difficult to detect and are too small to cause any damage. But now pharmaceutical companies are working to develop drugs that can knock out these and larger tumors by cutting off their blood supply. Called Angiogenesis Inhibitors, this class of drug was not available when this book was written, but it could be on the market in a few years' time. The

76

rationale behind these drugs is that if angiogenesis can be stopped, so can the growth of a tumor.

For as long as angiogenesis can be prevented, a tumor will stop growing. And if angiogenesis can be prevented permanently, this is virtually the same as total remission.

Micronutrients in Plant Foods May Inhibit Angiogenesis Now

A more natural way to induce angiogenesis—available to everyone at the present—may be to eat 15 or so servings of fruits and vegetables each day. IB #4 describes how micronutrients in plant-based foods may block angiogenesis in small tumors in the body and halt further growth.

These plant micronutrients may also inhibit angiogenesis in metastasized cells. If you have already had cancer, you can statistically reduce the risk of a recurrence by adopting IBs #3, #4, #6 and #8 and staying with them permanently for life—with your doctor's permission, of course.

No one is claiming that plant-based foods can cure cancer but strong indications point to the fact that angiogenesis may be inhibited by certain phytomins in foods that grow on plants. Some nutritionists are already calling these phytomins Angiogenesis Inhibitors.

A very recent study by John Pezzuto, Ph.D. at the University of Illinois, Chicago found that a substance in grapes called *resveratrol* helps keep cells from becoming cancerous and may help prevent the spread of malignancies. Eating grapes every day is the best source of resveratrol.

In other words, phytomins with antitumor qualities (carotenoids, flavonoids, indoles, isoflavones, protease inhibitors and sulphur compounds, all described in IB #4) are believed

77

capable of keeping carcinoma in situ dormant for years or decades. Since carcinoma in situ is rarely recognized by immune system cells, it places no burden on the immune system, and most people would then die of something else.

Phyto Estrogens May Prevent Breast and Prostate Cancer

Phyto estrogens are estrogens found in plant-based foods, particularly in soybeans and flaxseed, but also in citrus rind, seeds, fruits, whole grains and leafy green vegetables. Although study results are preliminary, it is believed that phyto estrogens in these foods may cancel out or neutralize the body's own estrogens.

Pure estrogen, which exists naturally in the body, is the female sex hormone. Exposure to the body's own estrogen over several decades may help promote breast cancer. Likewise, decades of exposure to testosterone, the body's natural male hormone, may also help promote prostate cancer. Both breast and prostate cancers are considered hormone-related.

Phyto estrogens are weak by comparison with body estrogen, but a person who eats several servings of foods rich in phyto estrogens each day may experience a significantly reduced risk of developing breast or prostate cancer. While clinical studies remain to be done, strong epidemiological evidence points to one indisputable fact: that people who eat a plant-based diet have a dramatically reduced incidence of breast or prostate cancer.

A word of caution: While eating plant micronutrients may help slow or even stop the growth of a small tumor, it should not be misconstrued as a substitute for seeing your doctor should any symptoms of cancer appear.

78

The Worst Way to Boost Your Immunity

Now that gene and other tests can predict your risk of developing various types of cancer, being forewarned about increased susceptibility could help you prevent it. However, merely having a gene susceptible for colon, breast or ovarian cancer is no guarantee you will actually develop the disease. Test results are far from being 100 percent dependable. And a favorable result showing low risk for, say, colon cancer could create a false sense of security, causing a person to follow a high-risk diet and lifestyle that could promote colon cancer after all.

Perhaps the worst way to save your immune system from having to battle cancer is to have a breast, colon or other body part surgically removed because a gene test shows you are susceptible to cancer in one of these sites. Yet prophylactic removal of healthy breasts or colons is fairly common in people with a family history of cancer in these locations.

Curiously, few physicians seem to counsel these patients to follow a diet and lifestyle that would reduce the risk of these cancers ever occurring.

HOW TO RECOGNIZE AND PREVENT SOME COMMON TYPES OF CANCER

Whether you have already had cancer and are worried about a recurrence, or a gene test or family history has predicted susceptibility for a specific cancer type, or your lifestyle and diet suggest that you might be at risk for a certain type of cancer, here are the facts to help you evaluate your risk of developing the most common forms of cancer. Each

79

review also defines risk factors you should eliminate and steps you can adopt to prevent each type of cancer from ever developing.

Prostate Cancer

Prostate cancer is the most common type of cancer in men. Growth of this cancer is stimulated by testosterone, the male sex hormone. One American male in five develops prostate cancer, and it strikes men most often in their sixties and seventies. But approximately 30 percent of all American men over 50 have activated cancer cells in the prostate, and microscopic clusters of prostate cancer cells are quite common in men in their thirties. Prostate cancer is classified as:

1. Low-grade if growth is quite slow.
2. High-grade if growth is rapid and virulent.

Medical care is essential in either case, but many doctors nowadays prefer "watchful waiting"—that is, observation without treatment—for low-grade cancer in older men. Further growth of low-grade prostate cancer may be retarded by using some of the Immune Boosters in this book. A combination of IBs #3, #4 ,#6 and #8 may well slow growth to the point where a significant tumor never develops. For many older men this is equivalent to a cure. Even though you use the Immune Booster techniques in this book to inhibit further growth, you must do so in cooperation with your doctor if prostate cancer has been diagnosed.

In any case, see a doctor if you have symptoms such as interrupted urine flow; difficulty starting or stopping urination; the need to urinate frequently, especially at night; blood in the urine; or a chronic pain in the lower back, upper thighs or pelvis. An annual digital rectal exam is usually recommended for men over 40 plus an annual Prostate Specific Antigen (PSA) test for men over 50. Perhaps by now there are new and improved tests.

The Causes of Prostate Cancer

A *High-Fat Diet.* Many of the same foods that promote free radicals have been identified as causing prostate cancer. These gremlin foods are described in IB #3: Cut Back on Foods That Cripple Your Immune System.

For instance, the death rate from prostate cancer is highest in countries where men consume the most fat (Sweden, Denmark, Canada, U.S.A.) and lowest in countries where the least fat is eaten, notably Southeast Asia. Men in Western countries have many times the risk of prostate cancer than do men in much of Asia. Prostate cancer growth is boosted by the hormone testosterone, and the more fat a man eats, the higher his testosterone level.

Race. Black American males have a 37 percent greater risk of developing prostate cancer than whites. The difference is believed to be due to poorer health habits among black men rather than to any genetic reason.

Sedentary Living. A survey of 13,000 men with an average age of 44, made at the Cooper Clinic in Dallas between 1970 and 1989, found that men who performed the most aerobic exercise had the lowest rate of prostate cancer.

Those who did the most exercise (and burned 3,000 or more calories per week) showed a rate of prostate cancer 70 percent lower than men who exercised least. Those who performed a moderate level of exercise (and burned 2,000 or more calories per week) reduced their risk by 25 percent.

Similar studies around the world all showed the same

81

pattern of results. Some researchers believe that intense exercise prevents prostate cancer by reducing testosterone levels. In lab animals, those with the lowest testosterone levels are least likely to develop prostate cancer. Being 20 pounds or more overweight, or having a BMI over 25, has also been linked to prostate cancer.

Meat. Considerable evidence indicates that a high intake of meat is associated with prostate cancer, and fat in the meat may not be the only cancer promoter. Some researchers suspect it could be a high level of animal protein. Dairy products are also high in animal protein. Interestingly, dairy foods are rare in Asia where prostate cancer incidence is low.

Ways to Prevent Prostate Cancer

Prostate cancer is almost entirely preventable through a combination of plant-based foods and daily exercise.

Eat a Low-Fat Diet High in Fruits, Vegetables and Other Foods That Grow on Plants. Animal studies at Memorial Sloan-Kettering Cancer Center, New York, showed that it was difficult to grow prostate cancer in mice fed a low-fat diet. The study, reported in the *Journal of the National Cancer Institute* (Oct. 4, 1995), revealed that when human prostate cancer cells were transferred to mice, they grew only half as fast in mice fed a diet containing 21 percent of calories from fat as in mice fed a diet in which 40 percent of calories were derived from fat.

A summary of the best advice is to eat a diet containing at least nine servings of fruits and vegetables (a half cup equals one serving) and one or more servings of soy products daily plus 10 servings of tomato products per week, especially tomato sauce prepared with a small amount of olive oil. A daily serving of grapes should also be included. Together

82

with whole grains, beans and a few nuts and seeds, such a diet should easily provide 30 to 35 grams of fiber daily.

An important study at Harvard Medical School, reported in the *Journal of the National Cancer Institute* (vol. 87, no. 23, 1995), on 48,000 male health care professionals evaluated the results of eating 46 different kinds of fruits and vegetables over the years 1986 to 1992.

Of the 46 plant foods, the lowest incidence of prostate cancer occurred in men who consumed a high intake of tomatoes or tomato products. Men who ate 10 or more servings of tomato sauce or paste showed 35 to 45 percent less risk of prostate cancer than men eating the Standard American Diet, while men eating tomatoes 4 to 7 times a week had a 22 percent reduction in risk.

The greatest risk reduction—45 percent—occurred in men who ate tomato sauce cooked in a small amount of olive oil. The tomato products can be part of any fat-free dish consisting solely of plant foods. Researchers believe that olive oil enhances absorption of the phytomin lycopene (described in IB #4: The One Diet That Does It All).

When one or more daily servings of soy products is also eaten, prostate cancer risk appears to be reduced still more. Indications are that this combination, in addition to a diet high in plant foods (particularly grapes) and daily exercise, may retard or even block further growth in a small tumor already in place. (Caution: This is not a substitute for medical diagnosis and evaluation.)

Try, also, to consume eight glasses of water or other nonalcoholic liquids daily. Avoid alcohol entirely, and cut out all foods that promote free radicals (described in IBs #3 and #4). Such a diet should gradually restore your BMI to normal and also prevent heart disease and diabetes.

Exercise. A brisk daily walk for 30 minutes or more, or a

83

comparable amount of other aerobic exercise such as bicycling or swimming, will help prevent further activation of prostate cancer cells.

Breast Cancer

One in every eight American women will develop this hormone-related cancer during her lifetime. Although the mortality rate is dropping, the number of cases is increasing, especially among black women. Breast cancer is the second leading cause of death in women.

Most people believe that breast cancer is caused by chemotherapy, food additives, hormone treatment, pesticides, pollution and radiation—all things which appear to be beyond our control. However, this is not true. Women have almost total control over the leading causes of breast cancer if they are willing to do what's required.

Causes of Breast Cancer

Family History. Breast cancer seems to run in families, but the explanation may be that the entire family ate the same diet, drank the same amount of alcohol, followed the same sedentary lifestyle and smoked cigarettes.

Age, Race. Only one woman in a hundred develops breast cancer before age 45, but the rates climb steadily thereafter. Caucasian and black women have a higher risk than Asian and Amerindian women.

Hormones. Breast cancer is due, at least in part, to naturally occurring hormones such as estrogen and progesterone. Obesity, which produces more hormones in the body, is also associated with higher risk. A late pregnancy (after age 34),

84

early menarche or never having a child may also increase the risk. Being raised on formula instead of being breast-fed as an infant may also increase risk. Alcohol consumption, even at a low level, is a proven risk.

Diet. Lack of fruits, vegetables and other plant foods in the diet significantly increases the risk.

How to Prevent Breast Cancer

Eat a Low-Fat Diet of Foods That Grow on Plants. Some researchers have failed to find a link between breast cancer and dietary fat, but epidemiological studies from more than 100 countries have shown conclusively that breast cancer is lowest in countries where the least fat is eaten. Many women have cancer-initiated breast cells with receptors for estrogen. When body estrogen binds with these receptors, it may stimulate the process of transforming these cells into activated cancer cells.

If you must use cooking oils, substitute olive oil for such high-risk oils as polyunsaturated vegetables oils and partially hydrogenated vegetable oils. (These oils are prime promoters of free radicals and are described in IBs #3 and #6.) In any case, keep total fat intake below a maximum of 20 percent of all calories from fat.

In 1996, a Harvard School of Public Health study suggested that eating a variety of fruits and vegetables might cut the risk of breast cancer by at least 20 percent. Other sources have estimated that if you don't smoke or consume alcohol, eat any foods that promote free radicals, and instead eat an abundance of foods that grow on plants, and also exercise daily, you could easily cut the risk of breast cancer by 60 to 75 percent, or possibly more.

Cut Out Alcohol. A survey of studies found that women

85

who have one alcoholic drink per day have a risk of breast cancer 11 percent higher than women who consume only two to three drinks per week. Anything over four drinks a week increases the risk.

Stay Trim by Exercising Aerobically for at Least 35 Minutes Each Day. Women who do not exercise have a breast cancer risk 1.85 times greater than women who exercise.

Have Regular Medical Checkups. In women over 50, a mammogram and a clinical breast exam every 1 to 2 years can halve the risk of mortality from breast cancer.

Lung Cancer

Due almost entirely to cigarette smoking, lung cancer kills 159,000 Americans annually. Since the early 1900s, lung cancer has killed more American women than breast cancer, and it is now the leading cause of mortality in women over 35.

Activated cancer cells develop in the bronchial tubes where cigarette smoke is inhaled and spread into the lungs. Seventy percent of lung cancer cases are incurable by the time they are diagnosed, and most victims die within five years. Once established, lung cancer overwhelms the immune system and spreads rapidly. Yet most cases can be prevented, even in people who have been smoking for several years.

Causes of Lung Cancer

Cigarette smoking is responsible for 80 percent of all cases. Exposure to air pollution, arsenic, asbestos, radiation and radon are responsible for a small percentage of cases.

People who have had TB, who are exposed to second-hand smoke or who eat too few fruits and vegetables also have an above-average risk.

How to Prevent Lung Cancer

Stop Smoking Today, Right Now and Forever! Precancerous lesions often disappear after a person stops smoking.

Cut Out Alcohol! Alcoholic drinks of all types work synergistically with cigarette smoke to intensify cancer risk.

Eat an Abundance of Plant Foods. Spinach and other green leafy vegetables plus carrots and sweet potatoes all abound in carotene, a phytomin that reduces the risk of lung cancer. At the same time, cut out all foods that promote free radicals (described in IBs #3 and #6). And continue to eat this way for the rest of your life.

Colorectal Cancer

Approximately one American in twenty develops colorectal cancer. Almost all consume above-average amounts of foods that promote free radicals and exercise little. Nine out of ten cases can be cured if detected early, but if metastases occurs, fewer than 7 percent currently survive.

Causes of Colorectal Cancer

Meat. Strong indications point to a diet rich in red meat and saturated (animal) fat and low in fruits, vegetables and dietary fiber.

Family History. People whose relatives have had colorectal cancer are considered at higher risk. But since only one American in 300 is said to carry a gene that increases colo-

87

rectal cancer risk, it seems more likely that all members of a cancer-prone family grew up spurning exercise and eating the same high-fat foods that promote free radicals.

Gender. Women who have had breast cancer or cancer of the genital organs are believed to have a higher risk of colorectal cancer.

Obesity and Sedentary Living. Both are proven risk factors, partly because regular exercise helps speed up bowel transit time.

How to Prevent Colorectal Cancer

Eat a Plant-Based Diet High in Fiber. Colorectal cancer has been directly linked with frequency of defecation. People who eat a low-residue diet of white flour products and foods that promote free radicals may defecate only three to four times a week. Their bellies become a giant holding tank for the decomposed residue of 8 to 11 digested meals. When fecal matter moves this slowly through the bowels, microflora in the gut produce a variety of free radicals and potentially carcinogenic compounds that initiate and activate cells in the colon and rectum.

The solution is to switch to "The One Diet That Does It All" (see IB #4). Consisting entirely of plant-based foods high in insoluble fiber, these foods zap free radicals. They also speed up bowel transit time to just 18 to 24 hours. A person then defecates twice daily and holds only two to three digested meals in the colon.

The same Harvard Medical School study described under "Ways to Prevent Prostate Cancer" above also found that the same tomato products that slashed the risk of prostate cancer also significantly reduced the risk of colon cancer. The greatest protection occurred in men who ate a serving of tomato sauce or paste cooked in a few drops of olive oil on 10 occasions per week. The tomato products can be part of any fat-free dish consisting solely of plant-based foods. Eating a serving of grapes each day also helps prevent all types of cancer.

Exercise Abundantly. Begin a gradually increasing program of aerobic exercise by walking, cycling or swimming at a brisk pace for 35 minutes or more at least five days each week.

Nutritional Supplements. People with colorectal cancer often have a deficiency of folate and selenium. Though no proof exists that these nutrients prevent cancer, it wouldn't hurt to maintain normal levels of both by taking supplements (see IB #2).

Medical Checkups. Traditionally, most doctors have recommended a digital rectal examination annually starting at age 40. Beginning at age 50, a stool specimen should be checked annually for blood. Then every 4 years after age 50, doctors may perform a sigmoidoscopy examination of the lower colon. (You can also test yourself for blood in the stool by using a Hemocult card that detects tiny traces of blood. But it does not diagnose colorectal cancer.)

Nowadays, however, for people with no evidence of colon problems, many doctors are giving a single colonoscopy examination at age 55. Unless new symptoms appear, no other tests are given. Anyone who exercises regularly and eats a plant-based diet should have an extremely low risk of colorectal cancer.

Other Types of Cancer

Smoking or use of smokeless tobacco, alcohol consumption, physical inactivity and lack of fruits, vegetables and whole grains in the diet have been identified as the causes

89

of most types of cancer. This is particularly true of cancer of the esophagus, larynx and mouth and of the cervix, kidneys and stomach.

Cervical cancer, which may be caused by a virus, could be all but eliminated if women had a regular Pap test. Women who begin sexual activity at a young age and who have had numerous sexual partners are at highest risk.

Overian cancer usually occurs after age 50. Since it can grow for years without symptoms—and be a constant burden on the immune system—it's prudent to have a regular pelvic exam if symptoms are suspected (bloating and swelling in the abdomen, indigestion, nausea and loss of appetite and weight). Elevated cholesterol levels also increase the risk of ovarian cancer. Cholesterol levels are easily lowered by adopting a low-fat, plant-based diet high in fiber (see IB #4). In a small study, a deficiency of selenium was associated with increased risk for ovarian cancer.

NATURAL WAYS TO CANCER-PROOF YOUR BODY

Currently, almost one American in three develops cancer at some time in life. Some sources now estimate that by 2005, two of every five Americans will develop cancer. The top ten cancer sites in women are the lung, breast, colorectal, ovary, pancreas, lymphoma, uterus, leukemia, liver and brain. The top ten in men are the lung, prostate, colorectal, pancreas, lymphoma, leukemia, esophagus, liver, stomach and bladder. Among ethnic groups in the United States, black men have the highest incidence of cancer and the highest mortality.

Whether through surgery, chemotherapy, drugs, radiation or bone marrow transplant, treatment can be extremely unpleasant and can destroy a person's quality of life. Each of these treatments also suppresses the immune system.

Clearly, the way to protect our immune systems is to prevent cancer up front. That is, to halt it by health-building diet and lifestyle habits long before it can ever challenge and overload our immune systems. And this isn't just pie in the sky.

According to the American Cancer Society, we can do exactly that. In an advisory released in September 1996, the society recommended that to prevent cancer, you should:

1. Choose most of the foods you eat from plant sources. Eat five or more servings of fruits and vegetables and breads, cereals, grains, rice or beans several times a day.

2. Limit intake of high-fat foods, especially meat and other foods from animal sources.

3. Exercise aerobically for at least 30 minutes on most days of the week. Reduce your BMI to 25 or below.

4. Limit consumption of alcoholic beverages or, better, don't drink at all.

This advice from one of the nation's leading health advisory agencies just about confirms everything else in this chapter. Cut out smoking and follow the society's guidelines, and you will not only prevent cancer but win back much of the immune power you had in your youth.

CHAPTER FOUR

How to Use This Book to Maximize Your Immunity

The role of the immune system is to protect us against cancer and infections. So it's not surprising that the main focus of this book is about preventing cancer. You will probably find more valid and authentic advice about cancer prevention within these pages than in almost any book written thus far about preventing cancer.

In fact, most books I have read about preventing cancer zero in on dietary supplements but completely overlook the far more powerful anticancer nutrients in fruits and vegetables and the tremendous cancer-preventing powers of exercise and a positive attitude.

The same is true of most other factors that boost immunity. Being overweight impairs the immune system on both the physical and the psychological levels. But most books about weight loss deal only with diet. Certainly, obesity can be curbed by diet. But to really reduce your weight to normal requires exercise and an attitude committed to overcoming obesity for good.

So don't be surprised to find more valid and authentic advice about losing weight within these pages than in most books that are entirely devoted to weight loss. This book also covers more about the amazing benefits of micronutrients in plant foods than almost any other book on that subject.

This is because immuno-suppression is a whole-person dysfunction, and it takes a whole-person approach to really supercharge it.

SO WHAT DOES HOLISTIC REALLY MEAN?

"Holistic" or "whole-person" are some of the most misused terms in the natural health field. Many of us believe that taking an herbal medicine or a dietary supplement is holistic. It isn't! Nor is merely eating lots of fruits and vegetables.

Holistic or whole-person implies putting the combined powers of body, mind and nutrition to work simultaneously. When we use one Immune Booster that works on the physical level, one on the psychological level and one on the nutritional level, we are using a truly holistic or whole-person approach.

It's like comparing the effect of a single musical instrument, which may render a magnificent solo, with the combined power and effect of all the instruments in a symphony orchestra playing in harmony.

Not surprisingly, then, this book recommends a whole-person approach, and it describes 18 natural immune-boosting thera-

93

pies, each featured under chapters covering the physical, psychological and nutritional approaches.

To help you get started quickly, here is a brief guide to the Immune Boosters you should consider for various circumstances and conditions.

If You're Looking for a Quick Fix

If you believe in quick fixes, turn to these Immune Boosters:

IB #1: *Herbs That Help Your Immune System.* The effect of most herbs is mild, but for a week or two they may help revitalize your immunity.

IB #2: *Restore Your Immune Power with Vitamins and Minerals.* Many people have a nutritional deficiency that impairs the performance of their immunity. Taking supplementary vitamins and minerals may help to overcome the deficiency and restore your immune system to normal functioning.

IB #15: *Beat Immuno-Suppression with Laughter Therapy.* Scientific tests have proved that this "mother of quick fixes" can boost your immunity by a measurable amount in just 30 minutes.

With a little more time and effort, you could add:

IB #3: *Cut Back on Foods That Cripple Your Immune System.* This action-step requires only that you cut out "bad guy" foods that harm your health. The same counterproductive foods also contribute to cancer, heart disease, obesity and a host of other human ailments.

IB #4: The One Diet That Does It All. By replacing the "bad guy" foods in your diet with the "good guy" foods in this Immune Booster, you can help your immunity and begin feeling better in just a few days.

If Your Goal Is to Prevent Cancer

After thoroughly reading Chapter 3: How to Stop Cancer Up Front; Before It Overloads the Immune System, focus on these Immune Boosters:

IB #3: Cut Back on Foods That Cripple Your Immune System

IB #4: The One Diet That Does It All

IB #5: The 8-Step Weight-Loss and Immune-Boosting Program

IB #6: Boost Your Immunity by Eating Lean

IB #8: Unlock Your Immune Power with Aerobic Exercise

IB #9: The Stronger Your Muscles, the Stronger Your Immunity

IB #13: Sleep Your Way to Stronger Immunity

IB #15: Beat Immuno-Suppression with Laughter Therapy

IB #16: Melt Away Stress and Tension with Relaxation Training

IB #17: Therapeutic Imagery: Create Your Own Neuropeptides and Talk to Your Immune System in a Language It Can Understand

IB #18: Defuse Depression with Cognitive Positivism

If Being Overweight Could Be Suppressing Your Immunity

Carrying excess body weight physically impairs immuno-competence while it also impairs your self-image and self-esteem. In turn, these subjective factors then intensify the damage to your immunity. If this sounds like your problem, look up these Immune Boosters:

IB #3: Cut Back on Foods That Cripple Your Immune System

IB #4: The One Diet That Does it All

IB #5: The 8-Step Weight-Loss and Immune-Boosting Program

IB #8: Unlock Your Immune Power with Aerobic Exercise

IB #9: The Stronger Your Muscles, the Stronger Your Immunity

If You're Concerned about an Allergy or an Autoimmune Disease

These conditions are caused when the immune system becomes confused, disoriented or distorted and then mal-functions. Autoimmune diseases, such as rheumatoid arthritis, occur when instead of defending the body, the immune system attacks cells and cartilage in our joints instead.

Space prevents in-depth discussion of autoimmune diseases in this book. Instead, I recommend your reading an earlier but still accurate book in this series entitled *18 Natural Ways to Stop Arthritis Now,* available through your bookseller or direct from Keats Publishing.

For more about allergies and how to prevent them, turn to:

IB #14: Allergies: What to Do When the Immune System Errs

II You Don't Know What May Be Compromising Your Immunity

Let's say you're exercising and eating a healthy diet but still get frequent colds and infections. In that case, read the following Immune Boosters. One or more of the topics they cover may be suppressing your immunity.

IB #7: Don't Let Food-Borne Infections Overload Your Immunity

IB #10: Pushing Yourself Too Hard Physically Can Suppress Your Immunity

IB #11: How to Stop Common Infections from Assaulting the Immune System

IB #12: Protect Your Immune System from Photo Damage

IB #13: Sleep Your Way to Stronger Immunity

IB #15: Beat Immuno-Suppression with Laughter Therapy

IB #18: Defuse Depression with Cognitive Positivism

If You Think Depression Is Suppressing Your Immunity

Depression or anxiety can literally devastate your immunity. If you constantly feel blue, look up the following Immune Boosters:

IB #8: Unlock Your Immune Power with Aerobic Exercise

IB #18: Defuse Depression with Cognitive Positivism

If Stress Seems to Be Weakening Your Immune System

Stress can erode our immunity more than any other single factor. If you suspect that stress is the culprit, read Chapter 7: The Psychological Approach: Don't Let Stress Trash Your Immunity. Then use the Immune Boosters below to help defuse your stress:

IB #8: Unlock Your Immune Power with Aerobic Exercise

IB #13: Sleep Your Way to Stronger Immunity

IB #15: Beat Immuno-Suppression with Laughter Therapy

IB #16: Melt Away Stress and Tension with Relaxation Training

IB #17: Therapeutic Imagery: Create Your Own Neuropeptides and Talk to Your Immune System in a Language It Can Understand

IB #18: Defuse Depression with Cognitive Positivism

If You Believe That Sleep Deficiency Is Sapping the Vigor of Your Immunity

Some researchers are suggesting that sleep is an integral part of our immune system and that failing to get sufficient sleep can ravage our immuno-competence. If lack of sleep is your problem, look up the Immune Boosters below:

IB #8: Unlock Your Immune Power with Aerobic Exercise

IB #13: Sleep Your Way to Stronger Immunity

IB #16: Melt Away Stress and Tension with Relaxation Training

What to Do about Frequent Colds and Infections

A weakened immune system has a harder time fighting off colds and infections. Be sure to read Chapter 2: Understanding Immunity: How the Immune System Works and Why. Then check out these Immune Boosters:

IB #1: Herbs That Help Your Immune System

IB #2: Restore Your Immune Power with Vitamins and Minerals

IB #7: Don't Let Food-Borne Infections Overload Your Immunity

IB #8: Unlock Your Immune Power with Aerobic Exercise

IB #10: Pushing Yourself Too Hard Physically Can Suppress Your Immunity

IB #11: How to Stop Common Infections from Assaulting the Immune System.

IB #12: Protect Your Immune System from Photo Damage

The listings just given are merely guidelines to direct you to the most helpful Immune Boosters for each ailment or dysfunction. As a result, the lists themselves may not always be holistic. Not all listings include Immune Boosters that work on the physical, psychological and nutritional levels. So for a completely holistic approach, I'm leaving it up to you to add whichever other Immune Boosters you feel are most appropriate.

Adopt a Single Immune Booster at a Time

Right off, you're probably wondering how you can possibly adopt half a dozen different Immune Booster techniques at the same time, let alone where you'll find time to practice them.

Don't worry!

Instead, merely adopt the one Immune Booster that seems most vital. Practice it each day until you can do it in a minimum of time. With a few days' practice, for example, IB #16 can take you into a state of deep and restful relaxation within 2.5 minutes, and often less.

Once you have used them, most of the nutrition action-steps take little extra time. And the same is true of most other Immune Boosters. It may take you a few sessions to learn how to do them. But once mastered, they become second nature.

Yes, a few exceptions do exist. A 35-minute aerobic exercise program will always take 35 minutes. And you may need extra time for sleep. But these are an essential part of any healthy lifestyle. Failing to exercise or to get sufficient sleep is tantamount to throwing away your life and health.

A MODEST PROPOSAL

Several readers of earlier books in this series have found an easy way to adopt some or all of the *18 Natural Ways* into their lives. Their solution has been to make health their hobby. Their food, their physical and mental recreation and even their vacations are all built around the wise health choices described in these books.

Rather than watching TV, they have built their leisure around more healthful and wholesome activities. For example, they suggest bicycling, brisk canoe paddling or rowing, jogging, swimming, tennis and walking; playing basketball, soccer or volleyball; cross-country skiing or skating; practicing yoga; or performing a strength-building workout at the local gym.

For something more intellectually creative and stimulating than TV, consider taking up painting, reading literature or writing, learning to play a musical instrument; teaching yourself more about sciences like astronomy, biology, chemistry or cosmology; learning to use a computer and roaming the Internet; or taking adult-education classes in these subjects and perhaps learning a new language.

Making love or laughing for half an hour is far more enjoyable than watching most TV shows. And consider taking back control of your food by spurning restaurant eating. Eat at home instead on plant-based foods purchased in the produce department of your local supermarket.

By making health your hobby, you can still thrive in the modern world without letting it sabotage your immunity.

101

CHAPTER FIVE

The Nutritional Approach: Eating for Peak Immunity

In one way or another, almost everything we eat helps either to boost or to suppress our immunity. The Immune Boosters in this section help you separate the "good guy" foods from the "bad guys" and they steer you towards making healthy food choices. The nutritional approach is also concerned with stopping cancer and infections up front before they can overload and suppress the immune system.

Right off, you can probably jump-start your immune system with the herbs in IB #1 or the vitamin-mineral supplements in IB #2. Vitamins D and E and the minerals selenium and zinc may prove to be a fountain of youth for aging immune cells.

But to really supercharge your immune system you'll need to read about phytomins, the most exciting disease-fighting nutrients discovered in modern times. Compelling new research has revealed that foods which grow on plants are chockful of disease-fighting chemicals called *phytomins*. These include powerful cancer inhibitors like glutathione, isoflavones and lycopene as well as fiber and antioxidants. All these nutrients help the immune system fight and overcome disease. They're described in detail in IB #4.

By contrast, IB #3 identifies a whole class of foods high in fat and low in fiber that work to cripple the immune system. Almost one-third of cancer is caused by these foods (as well as heart disease and other degenerative diseases that kill older Americans). Then IB #6 steers you through the maze of food traps that exhort you to overeat fat and sugar.

Yet being overweight has been identified as the single greatest immuno-suppressant on the nutritional scene. For starters, the Immune Boosters expose the futility of calorie-reducing fad diets. Instead, IB #5 presents a revolutionary new no-nonsense weight loss plan endorsed by almost every health advisory agency and university medical research center in America.

When combined with regular exercise and a positive attitude, these Immune Boosters offer a completely holistic way to supercharge your immunity through the nutritional approach.

IMMUNE BOOSTER #1: Herbs That Help Your
Immune System

Herbs may not always boost the immune system directly. But researchers in pharmacognosy, the scientific study of herbs, have found that scores of herbs have a powerful anti-

103

microbial action that helps the immune system destroy invading bacteria, fungi and viruses.

Yet it is often the phytomin content of herbs that explains their therapeutic qualities. Many drugs are manufactured from herbs. Other herbs are so rich in antioxidants and anticarcinogens that drug companies are constantly working to synthesize and patent them.

Meanwhile, hundreds of animal and lab studies have demonstrated that many herbs exhibit powerful disease-prevention qualities.

Each of the herbs described below was selected for its ability to help the immune system overcome cancer or infections.

Because much of the herbal market is unregulated and manufacturers often make claims that have not been substantiated, I recommend shopping for herbs at a store managed by someone who is thoroughly familiar with herbs and what they can really accomplish.

Caution: While some herbs may help prevent cancer or infections, they are not intended as a substitute for clearly needed medical treatment.

NATURAL IMMUNE BOOSTERS

A number of herbs are actually nature's own Immune Boosters. They include the following:

Echinacea (Purple Coneflower)

Pronounced ek-ee-nay-see-a, this popular garden herb is widely prescribed by herbalists to inhibit the symptoms of minor viral or bacterial infections such as colds, fever blisters or influenza. Some 25 small studies have found it an effective general immune system stimulant. For example, echinacea works by inhibiting bacteria from secreting the enzyme hyacuronidase that helps them sneak into the body through the membranes of skin, nose or throat. Echinacea also appears to be toxic to most viruses.

Several studies have reported that echinacea boosts production of complement and stimulates activity of T-cells. While echinacea lacks the power to halt a major infection, it can be used to complement antibiotic medical treatment.

Echinacea is widely available in capsules, pills and tinctures, all made from the roots of one or more varieties of the echinacea plant. Many herbalists believe that an alcohol or liquid extract is the most effective form.

Caution: Echinacea loses effectiveness if used daily for more than two weeks. It should not be used if you have an impaired immune function or an allergy to the sunflower family or if you suffer from an autoimmune disease such as lupus or rheumatoid arthritis.

Goldenseal (Hydrastis canadensis)

Many herbalists believe that goldenseal is a powerful immuno-stimulant because it dilates arteries leading to the spleen. As blood flow to the spleen increases, the spleen is believed to release compounds that stimulate the activity of macrophages.

In conjunction with standard medical treatment, goldenseal has proved an effective complementary medicine for treating infections such as *Candida albicans*, chlamydia, salmonella, staphylococcus and streptococcus. An alcohol extract of goldenseal is considered the most dependable.

Licorice Root

Because it contains glycyrrhizin, an acid believed to turn on interferon production by the immune system, herbalists often prescribe licorice root to treat a wide range of infections. Licorice root is certainly effective against fever blisters and when used in conjunction with medical treatment, it may stimulate the immune system to help fight *Candida albicans*, bronchitis, pharyngitis, pneumonia, staphylococcus and streptococcus.

Licorice root also contains phytomins with properties similar to those of the flavonoids found in soybeans. Dr. Herbert Pierson, an expert on phyto chemicals, has suggested that licorice root might inactivate estrogen in women. This property might then enable licorice root to prevent or retard the growth of hormone-related cancers such as those of the breast or prostate. Some herbalists also claim that the glycyrrhizic acid in licorice root may inhibit onset of prostate cancer by retarding conversion of the male hormone testosterone into the cancer promoter hydrotestosterone.

Licorice root is obtained by boiling the root of the licorice plant *Glycyrrhiza glabra*. It is not the same as the licorice used in confections or candy. To take licorice root, you simply eat a small amount. Because eating 2 to 3 ounces daily for a week or more may cause imbalances in body chemistry, including hypertension or even heart rhythm aberrations, consumption should be kept to 2.5 ounces or less per day. Anyone with heart disease or hypertension, or who is taking diuretics or heart drugs, should not take licorice root at all.

NATURAL ANTIDEPRESSANTS

Although they do not directly elevate immunity, the two natural antidepressant herbs described below certainly deserve inclusion. The reason, of course, is that depression is one of the most powerful immuno-suppressants in existence.

St. John's Wort (Hypericum)

More than twenty double-blind studies in Europe, involving more than 1,600 participants, have clearly demonstrated the effectiveness of St. John's Wort in relieving mild-to-moderate depression, anxiety, apathy and low self-esteem.

In one study of 84 people in Austria, for example, the 42 people in the study group each took 300 mg of St. John's Wort extract 3 times a day for one month. All 42 participants reported a strong uplift in mood while only 29 percent of those in the 42-member control group did. Several other European studies found St. John's Wort extract just as effective as several popular antidepressant drugs.

Researchers in Germany report that St. John's Wort relieves mild depression by breaking up amines that destroy mood-elevating brain chemicals. St. John's Wort benefits only mild-to-moderate depression, not moderate-to-severe depression. Mild-to-moderate depression is classified as the level at which symptoms do not intefere with daily living.

The herb is sold as a drug in Germany but in the United States is classified as a dietary supplement and is available in the form of capsules, dried leaves, liquid tablets, powder, oil or tea. Whichever form you buy, the label should state the hypericin content.

For best results, use only an extract of St. John's Wort

standardized to contain 0.3 percent (one-third of 1 percent) hypericum and take it at the dosage of 300 mg three times a day. Never take more than 900 mg per day and never take it close to bedtime. If you are taking any medication, check with your physician before taking St. John's Wort.

Benefits should appear about 3 weeks after you begin taking St. John's Wort. While taking the herb, avoid foods high in tyramine such as red wine and cheese.

Gingko Biloba

Though best known for its ability to relieve asthma, gingko biloba has also been shown to uplift mood.

In one study, 40 elderly men and women with depression, who had failed to respond to standard antidepressant drugs, were each given 80 mg of gingko biloba extract three times a day. A similar group received a placebo.

Eight weeks later, the depression level in the study group had dropped by 66 percent compared with only 4 percent in the study (placebo) group. Other studies have shown that gingko biloba has enhanced the effectiveness of several common antidepressant drugs.

Gingko biloba should be standardized to contain 24 percent gingko flavoglycosidise (herterosides) and 6 percent terpenoid taken in a dosage of 40 to 80 mg three times a day.

IMMUNE BOOSTER #2: Restore Your Immune Power with Vitamins and Minerals

---

Brenda always seemed to catch everything that was going around. Minor cuts on her fingers seemed to take an age to heal. And whenever she spent a day outdoors, painful fever blisters would break out on Brenda's lips.

When a friend noticed Brenda's diet—an appalling mix of junk food, white bread, hamburgers and coffee—she urged Brenda to start taking a multiple vitamin-mineral supplement. She also persuaded Brenda to begin eating three fruits and five vegetables each day.

Sick of the constant infections, Brenda agreed. For several weeks, she showed no improvement. Then, gradually, Brenda began to feel better. Weeks went by and she did not catch a cold or develop fever blisters A cut on her finger healed in 48 hours.

When it became apparent that nutrition really was working, Brenda's enabling effect kicked in. Fired with new energy, she cut out all meat, poultry, eggs, fried foods and all but nonfat dairy foods from her diet, and she replaced them with six or more servings of fruits and 12 or more servings of vegetables each day.

The friend told us that in the two years that followed, Brenda suffered from only a single cold—from which she fully recovered in just four days.

No, Brenda didn't supercharge her immune system—although that's what it felt like. What really happened was that she restored her badly suppressed immune function to normal. Like millions of other Americans, Brenda's diet was sadly deficient in several key nutrients that are essential to optimal functioning of the immune system.

Nutritional Deficiencies Are Responsible for Millions of Cases of Suppressed Immunity

Several large surveys have confirmed that many Americans 55 and over have compromised immune systems due to a deficiency of one, two or more key nutrients in the diet. Several studies have shown that as many as three-fourths of all teenagers, pregnant women and older people may be getting only 60 to 70 percent of their daily vitamin and mineral requirements.

Anyone whose diet is built around the "bad guy" foods described in IB #3, who lives on the Standard American Diet or who eats few fruits, vegetables, beans and whole grains is likely to be deficient in several important nutrients. Further nutritional depletion is often caused by emotional stress or by taking certain prescription drugs, especially those for rheumatoid arthritis.

Add in the reduced ability to absorb and assimilate nutrients that occurs with advancing age, and these factors can drain the body's nutrient resources faster than the Standard American Diet can replenish them. So it's hardly surprising that millions of Americans have poorly stabilized immune systems.

This fact was confirmed in a 1995 study by John Blodgen, Ph.D., professor of preventive medicine and community health at New Jersey Medical School, Newark. He and his researchers found that when people aged 60 and over took a multiple vitamin-mineral supplement each day for one year, their immune response improved by a whopping 60 percent. Meanwhile, no change occurred in a control group taking a placebo.

Another important finding of this study was that older people benefited most from higher levels of vitamins and minerals than the current Recommended Daily Allowance (RDA). As growing evidence shows that these RDAs do not meet the nutritional needs of older Americans, more and more nutritionists are recommending that people over 60 take a multi that contains 200 percent of the RDA for most vitamins.

How to Restore Your Immunity to Normal

If you are functionally deficient in any vitamins and minerals essential to immune system health, you may jump-start your immune system in just a week or two by putting the missing nutrients back into your diet. For anyone with a nutritionally deficient immune system, this one step may restore immuno-competence to its normal vigorous level.

But don't confuse a normal level of immunity with a supercharged immune system. By using other Immune Boosters in this book, particularly those that use a psychological approach, you can send your immunity soaring to new, higher levels far above the normal range.

Such superhigh levels are rarely reached by taking megadoses of nutritional supplements. Once the nutritional needs of your immune system are met, the best way to help your immunity is by eliminating as many "bad guy" foods from your diet as you can and by including as many "good guy" foods as you possibly can.

("Bad guy" foods are described in IB #3 and "good guy" foods in IB #4.)

Plant Foods Are the Best Sources of Vitamins and Minerals

Along with many nutritionists, I recommend getting most of your vitamins and minerals from foods rather than from dietary supplements. That's because vitamins and minerals are most numerous in fruits, vegetables, whole grains, legumes, nuts and seeds—the same plant-based foods that are loaded with fiber and that abound with cancer-fighting nutrients called phytomins (see IB #4). Nutritional supplements, by contrast, lack any of the hundreds of antioxidants, other nutrients and substances such as fiber that are numerous in foods that grow on plants.

Provided you adopt the "One Diet That Does It All" described in IB #4, you are unlikely to experience any significant nutritional deficiency. However, if you eat no foods at all of animal origin—including eggs or dairy products—you should take a vitamin B12 supplement (best taken along with other B vitamins as part of a multi). And if you do not eat any dairy products at all, you would probably benefit from a daily calcium supplement that also contains magnesium and vitamin D.

In any case, it wouldn't hurt to take a multi once a day. And regardless of how packed with nutrients your foods are, it is almost impossible to consume sufficient vitamin E without eating a dangerously high level of fat. I therefore recommend that you take a daily vitamin E supplement as described below.

If you are not able to follow IB #4, or to eat at least four fruits and eight vegetables daily, plus several servings of whole grain breads, cereals and one or more servings of legumes, then you very definitely should take a full spectrum multiple vitamin-mineral supplement every day.

A Good Multi Needn't Cost a Fortune

Many supermarkets and discount stores offer quality multis at significant savings. The best multis may carry the abbreviation "USP" or the term "U.S. Pharmocopeia Quality" on the label. But no multi can provide all the nutrients that most people require. That's because our daily requirements of calcium, magnesium and vitamins C and E are simply too bulky to be compressed into any single pill. Be sure to buy these nutrients separately.

While a multi that supplies 100 percent of the RDA for vitamins A, C and the B-complex should restore vitality to a nutrient-deficient immune system, anyone over 55 might benefit even more by taking a multi that contains 200 percent of certain vitamins.

Because most nutrients work in synergy with other vitamins and minerals, and also with phytomins in plant foods, taking supplements of single vitamins may be a waste of money. For example, vitamins C and E and the mineral selenium work together, as do vitamin D and calcium and magnesium.

Can dietary supplements help boost your immune system? Since only we know exactly what we eat, we are probably the best judges of our nutritional shortfalls and needs. To help you evaluate your own nutritional needs, here is a brief profile of each of the key vitamins and minerals which, when deficient in the body, may severely suppress the immune system.

VITAMINS AND MINERALS

While all vitamins and minerals are needed for optimal health, certain ones help boost your immunity.

Vitamin A

A deficiency of vitamin A may impair production of IgA antibodies, it may inhibit the ability of all antibodies to lock on to antigens, and it may reduce the number of lympho-

113

cytes circulating in the bloodstream. Rather than take vitamin A in supplement form, I recommend eating plant foods that are rich in beta-carotene, a precursor of vitamin A.

For instance, eating a medium-sized carrot supplies about 20,000 IU of vitamin A, and the beta-carotene in the carrot is more readily absorbed. In tests, beta-carotene obtained from foods has increased base levels of T-helper and NK cells.

Supplements of beta-carotene are no longer recommended. Instead, tests have shown that we need to absorb the entire spectrum of 40 or more carotenoids, all of which are found in such plant foods as apricots, butternut squash, canteloupes, carrots, sweet potatoes and just about all fruits and vegetables that have a rich orange color, as well as in greens like broccoli, kale and spinach.

While it is possible to overdose on vitamin A, you cannot overdose on eating plant foods rich in beta-carotene. Be sure to avoid vitamin A supplements if pregnant.

B-Complex Vitamins

B-complex vitamins are rapidly depleted by stress and are often low in people with autoimmune diseases or with compromised immunity. A deficiency of B vitamins is also common among people who consume more than three alcoholic drinks daily, while 80 percent of people with depression have low levels of B vitamins (depression is a direct suppressor of immunity).

Foods rich in most B vitamins include whole grains, wheat germ, brewers yeast, avocadoes, sweet potatoes, cruciferous vegetables, bananas, peanuts and most beans. However, vitamin B12 exists only in foods of animal origin such as plain nonfat yogurt.

Like almost all other nutrients, B vitamins work far better in combination with other B vitamins than singly. Thus taking a full-spectrum B-complex supplement is far preferable to taking supplements of single B-vitamins. Any B-complex supplement should include 400 mg of folate, plus at least the RDA of B1 (thiamine), B2 (riboflavin), B3 (niacin), B5 (pantothenic acid), B6 (pyridoxin), and B12 (cobalamin).

Vitamin B6 (pyridoxin.)

Studies at HNRC found that a deficiency of B6 could lead to abnormal functioning of the immune system. These dysfunctions disappeared when B6 was reintroduced. Taking 2 mg per day (the daily value), was found to help boost immunity, but only in someone who had an actual deficiency.

Folic Acid or Folate

Adequate levels of this B vitamin are necessary to help the immune system defend the body against cervical cancer, especially when a person is infected with human papilloma virus. A deficiency of folic acid has also been associated with a higher risk of lung and colorectal cancer. People taking drugs for autoimmune diseases often develop a deficiency of folic acid. Low levels of folic acid are also believed to directly suppress the immune system. Good food sources of folic acid are beans, wheat germ, brewer's yeast, whole grain cereals, leafy green vegetables and broccoli. Nowadays some white flour products and breakfast cereals are also fortified with folate.

Vitamin C (Abscorbic Acid)

Because it helps to neutralize adrenal hormones, vitamin C is rapidly consumed by the body under stress. Since stress suppresses the immune system, remaining supplies of vitamin C in the body are then drawn on to bolster immunity. When a person under stress takes aspirin, or similar painkillers, a severe deficiency may develop. Moreover, millions of people with suppressed immunity eat few, if any, fruits or vegetables, the principal dietary sources of vitamin C.

The result is a widespread and common deficiency of vitamin C that impairs the performance of every cell in the body, including those of the immune system. This deficiency slows wound healing and increases the risk of infection.

A diet of "good guy" foods—that is, foods that grow on plants—will swiftly restore a vitamin C deficiency in most people. Besides this, the best solution is to take one 250 mg supplement of ascorbic acid (vitamin C) in the morning and another 12 hours later. Since 250 mg will saturate every cell in the body of an average-sized person, there is little need to take more.

Foods that are high in vitamin C include strawberries, kiwi fruit, freshly squeezed or frozen concentrate orange or grapefruit juice, cantaloupe or honeydew melons, green peppers, cooked Brussel sprouts, oranges or grapefruit, turnip greens, mangoes, cauliflower, broccoli, cabbage, sweet potatoes, collard greens, cruciferous vegetables, tomatoes and tomato juice and snowpeas. Since vitamin C is lost by processing or cooking in water, it's best to eat these foods raw, lightly steamed or microwaved.

If you eat fewer than seven servings of fruits and vegetables daily, you may benefit from taking a vitamin C supplement. Because it is water-soluble and cannot penetrate fatty cells where free radicals lurk, vitamin C by itself is not a strong

116

antioxidant. But it is believed to serve as a catalyst in reinforcing the potency of other antioxidants.

Many other health benefits have been claimed for supplements of vitamin C, from enhancing thymus function to increasing synthesis of interferon and improving protein synthesis. But, as always, this vitamin is far more powerful when it works in conjunction with the hundreds of other nutrients and phytomins found in foods that grow on plants.

Calcium and Vitamin D

Calcium and vitamin D help the immune system by significantly reducing the incidence of colon cancer. Recent clinical and lab studies indicate that it is the calcium that helps prevent colon cancer; but for the calcium to work, it must first be metabolized by vitamin D.

Several large studies have demonstrated that a daily intake of 1200 mg of calcium and 200 IU or more of vitamin D reduced the risk of colorectal cancer by 50 to 75 percent. But, the studies found, millions of Americans are deficient in both calcium and vitamin D.

A 1995 study at HNRC found that adults need more vitamin D than the RDA of 200 IU. To prevent degenerative diseases, researchers concluded that we need at least 400 IU and for slender, fair-skinned Caucasian or Asian women possibly as much as 800 IU.

Plain nonfat yogurt is an ideal source of dietary calcium, but, unlike milk, it is not fortified with vitamin D. Thus many nutritionists advise taking a vitamin D supplement of 400 IU daily. Alternatively, most health food stores carry supplements that supply 1500 to 1800 mg of calcium and 400 IU of vitamin D.

You may also obtain beneficial amounts of calcium by

eating more tofu, sesame seeds, dark green leafy vegetables or mackerel, sardines or salmon. Vitamin D may be generated by sunbathing for 20 minutes 3 times a week. However, due to a weakened ozone layer and risk of skin cancer, sunbathing is advisable in summer only before 10 A.M. and after 3 P.M. Note that sunblock or sunscreen prevents absorption of vitamin D.

Vitamin E

Vitamin E may be a fountain of youth for aging immune cells. A study by Ranjit Chandra, Ph.D., professor of immunology at the University of Newfoundland, found that when older people were given a supplement of 800 IU of vitamin E daily, their immune response became as vigorous as that of an average person 10 years younger.

Another study at HNRC in 1996 showed that when older people were given vitamin E supplements, their T-cell function improved. In yet another study, when mice were given the human equivalent of 400 IU of vitamin E daily, the mice showed much less age-related damage to their immune cells.

To start with, vitamin E is a potent antioxidant. But as with so many nutrients when used alone, its benefits seem limited. Studies show it is very effective in preventing heart disease but considerably less so in preventing cancer.

However, when taken in conjunction with vitamin C, vitamin E has significantly prevented death from all causes. In a 9-year study of 11,000 people in their late 60s, those who took vitamin E alone had 34 percent fewer deaths from all causes during the study, while those taking vitamins E and C together had 42 percent fewer deaths. The typical study participant took 200 to 400 IU of vitamin E and 250 to

1,000 mg of vitamin C daily. Vitamin C alone had no effect on mortality.

Vitamin E's effectiveness as an antioxidant is also boosted when taken in conjunction with a diet of plant-based foods rich in antioxidants such as broccoli, celery, dark green leafy vegetables, yellow-orange fruits and vegetables, wheat germ and whole grains. Vitamin E appears to act as a catalyst to spur on other antioxidants.

Because vitamin E is fat-soluble and found primarily in high-fat foods, it is difficult to absorb enough from food without incurring an undesirably high intake of fat. Instead, most nutritionists suggest taking a daily supplement of 200 to 400 IU in either natural or synthetic form. Vitamin E is best taken in a separate capsule rather than as part of a multivitamin supplement.

For best absorption, take your vitamin E supplement with the fattiest meal of the day or with an avocado or beans. Better still, place a few drops of olive or canola oil on an 1-inch square piece of bread and eat that with the vitamin E supplement. Or slice open the vitamin E capsule and squeeze out the contents on to the oil-soaked bread.

Foods that contain some vitamin E are almonds, asparagus, filberts, green leafy vegetables, olives, pure almond or peanut butter, sunflower seeds and wheat germ. *Caution:* Anyone taking blood-thinning drugs may experience complications when taking vitamin E.

Magnesium

An adequate intake of magnesium is essential to maintain a healthy immune system balance. But most Americans are actually deficient in this key mineral. In fact, many Americans who are overweight, whose lives are stressed or who take drugs for an autoimmune disease are often drained of magnesium and have a serious deficiency.

One reason is because the Standard American Diet supplies barely 40 percent of the average person's magnesium requirements. When stress hormones flood the body during periods of tension, magnesium is drained from all immune cells, lowering resistance to virus infections and leaving a person feeling tired and exhausted.

A daily supplement of 250 mg or more of magnesium soon relieves anxiety and improves sleep. As with so many nutrients, however, the benefits of magnesium are almost doubled when it is taken in conjunction with calcium. Combined calcium-magnesium-vitamin D supplements are available at all health food stores.

The current RDA for magnesium is 280 mg for women and 350 mg for men. You can boost your magnesium intake by eating bananas, beans, leafy green vegetables, nuts and wheat germ.

Selenium

An important trace mineral found in the soil, selenium functions as an antioxidant to prevent skin cancer and coronary artery disease. It appears to protect the DNA of skin cells from solar radiation. Some animal and human studies also claim that a deficiency impairs immunity and increases the risk of several common forms of cancer.

In Third World countries, wherever selenium levels are low, colorectal cancer increases. But in the United States, despite low selenium content in soils in the Pacific Northwest, the Great Lakes area and east of the Mississippi generally, few Americans have a deficiency because our foods are shipped in from across the nation.

Nonetheless, it's important to maintain an adequate intake of selenium as we age because the mineral helps regulate the enzyme glutathione peroxide, a powerful phytomin that prevents cancer and heart disease and retards the aging process. Glutathione levels in the bloodstream drop gradually with age.

However, a 1997 study by Larry C. Clark, Ph.D. of Arizona Cancer Center College of Medicine, University of Arizona, Tucson, found that taking a daily selenium supplement significantly reduced cancer incidence and mortality. Participants in the study were all from an area in the eastern United States with low selenium content in the soil. Each participant took 200 mcg of supplemental selenium daily for 4.5 years. Compared with the control group, study participants had a 37 percent reduction in cancer incidence and a 50 percent reduction in cancer mortality.

Of cancer cases diagnosed during the study, there were 63 percent fewer prostate cancers, 58 percent fewer colorectal cancers and 46 percent fewer lung cancers than in the control group. No cases of selenium toxicity occurred.

According to the *Journal of the American Medical Association*, Dr. Clark believes that selenium inhibits tumor growth through its antioxidant properties, its ability to alter carcinogenic metabolism, its effects on the endocrine and immune systems and its power to inhibit protein synthesis.

You can ensure an adequate intake of selenium by eating several servings of whole, unrefined grains and cereals daily plus Brazil and other nuts, broccoli, brown rice, cabbage, carrots, celery, cucumbers, garlic, lentils, onions, soybeans, spinach and wheat germ. Just to be sure, however, many health professionals are now taking a daily supplement of

200 mcg. Selenium works best in conjunction with vitamin E.

Zinc

Adequate zinc is essential for optimal T-cell activity and for forming antibodies. But taking zinc improves immune function only if you have a zinc deficiency. And many people do have a zinc deficiency, particularly men and women over 65. Tests have shown that the average American over 65 takes in only 6 to 9 mg of zinc daily from food, while the RDA is 12 mg for women and 15 mg for men.

This was confirmed in a recent study by Ananda Prasad, Ph.D. of Wayne State University, Detroit. Out of 188 elderly white women, all of whom were zinc-deficient, Prasad found indications of depressed immunity in 36 of the women. When the 36 were given 30 mg of zinc daily, their levels of thymulin and interleukin-1 bounded up—a clear indication of the increased ability of their immune systems to fight disease. Other surveys showed similar zinc deficiencies in overweight people and in people taking drugs for rheumatoid arthritis.

Signs of a zinc deficiency include wounds that take a long time to heal, diminished sensitivity to taste; and recurring infections. It's a fairly safe bet that many middle-aged and older men and women have at least a marginal deficiency of zinc, meaning that their immune systems are not quite up to par.

How about the much-publicized ability of zinc lozenges to alleviate cold symptoms? Some studies have found no benefit, while others showed that taking zinc lozenges shortened the number of days during which cold symptoms persisted. But study authors are still not certain whether zinc boosts the immune system and speeds up antibody production, or whether zinc is simply toxic to cold viruses.

In one recent study, 100 people who had developed colds in the past 24 hours were each given a zinc lozenge every two hours while awake. The lozenge-takers experienced only 4.5 days of cold symptoms compared with 7.5 days of symptoms in a control group who took a placebo. But 20 percent of the lozenge-takers experienced nausea and 50 percent found the lozenges either unpleasantly bitter or sour. (The lozenges in the study are sold under the brand name Cold-Eeze. Other lozenges may be chemically different.)

The RDA of zinc is 12 mg for women and more for those pregnant or breastfeeding. Men's RDA is 15 mg. Most multivitamin supplements supply 15 mg. If you take a zinc supplement, your multi should also supply 2 mg or more of copper daily, since zinc can impair the body's ability to absorb copper. Never take more than 30 mg of zinc daily on a long-term basis. Megadoses merely suppress immunity. Some dietary zinc can be obtained by eating whole or fortified grains, breads and cereals, as well as beans, peanuts and dairy products.

Other Nutrients That May Boost Immunity

Among other nutrients linked to immunity or to cancer prevention are proteolytic enzymes and modified citrus protein.

Researchers in Germany have found that proteolytic enzymes support the immune system by stimulating macrophage activity and by helping the body eliminate immune complex. Immune complex is the residue formed when antibodies lock on to and disable bacteria. Among proteolytic enzymes widely available in health food stores are pancreatic enzymes with bromelain, a mixture that may also help the immune system identify and recognize cancer cells.

A study of rats by researchers at Wayne State School of Medicine recently found that modified citrus protein appears to inhibit metastasis of prostate cancer and may also slow tumor growth. A nutrient extracted from citrus pulp, modified citrus protein clings to cancer cells so that they are more easily recognized by T-cells. While animal studies are only preliminary, the outlook appears promising for upcoming clinical studies on humans. This nutrient may be available as a dietary supplement in health food stores by now.

IMMUNE BOOSTER #3: Cut Back on Foods That Cripple Your Immune System

---

Few foods actually assault our immune system head on. But a whole class of foods works indirectly to cripple our immunity. What these foods have in common is that they are all promoters of free radicals. And free radicals are responsible for most of the hundreds or thousands of activated cancer cells that our bodies produce every day. To keep us free of cancer, every last one of these cells must be destroyed by our immune system each day. More, perhaps, than anything else, the daily task of destroying a huge number of unnecessary cancer cells frequently overloads and weakens our immune systems.

These cancer cells are unnecessary because they are largely caused by certain foods we eat. The more foods we eat that promote free radicals, the more cancer cells our bodies produce each day and the greater the burden on our immune system. Moreover, the same foods that promote free radicals also promote eye diseases, heart disease, hypertension, obesity, stroke and most of the age spots, skin discoloration and wrinkles that age us prematurely.

If you ever hope to boost your immunity, it's vital to know exactly which foods these are. And then to eat as few as possible or, better, to strictly avoid them all. When we do that, we can dramatically cut the number of new cancer cells that appear in our bodies each day

THE FOODS THAT HARM OUR IMMUNE SYSTEM MOST: THE GREMLIN FOODS THAT PROMOTE FREE RADICALS

Meat, especially red meat and sausage, luncheon meats or any meats or fish that are salted, pickled or smoked. Lean meat, as well as meat high in fat, is now considered to increase the risk of cancer—and the risk may be due as much to the protein content as to the fat. Meat singed or charred while barbecuing may contain additional carcinogens.

Saturated fat, primarily found in foods of animal origin and in dairy products (except nonfat). Coconut and palm oils also have a high content of saturated fat.

Polyunsaturated vegetable oils, primarily cooking oils such as corn, cottonseed, safflower, soybean and sunflower oils.

Partially hydrogenated vegetable oils (also known as trans-fatty acids). These manufactured oils abound in margarine and in almost every form of commercial baked goods, processed foods and breads.

Poultry.

Eggs.

125

All fried foods, including French fries and fried fish and seafood.

Molecular Wrecking Balls That Damage DNA

Free radicals are formed when molecules of saturated or polyunsaturated fats or partially hydrogenated vegetable oils are oxidized in the body and transformed into electrically charged particles, each containing an unpaired electron. Once in our cells, these unstable molecules set off a chain reaction that has electrons jumping from gene to gene in a domino effect along the double helix of a cell's DNA.

Repeated bombardment by free radicals first initiates a cell by making it cancer-prone. Further assaults by free radicals and carcinogens then activate the initiated cell, transforming it into a fully fledged cancer cell. If that cell isn't immediately destroyed by our immune system, it may go on to create a life-threatening tumor. Other free radicals change the basic structure of cholesterol in the arteries, forming plaque that can block the coronary arteries and cause a fatal heart attack.

Free radicals occur spontaneously in polyunsaturated vegetable oils. Although these oils do not become discolored or cloudy, they swiftly turn rancid after being exposed to air. Foods fried in these oils become potential time bombs loaded with free radicals. This is particularly true if the oil is reheated and used over and over, a common practice in many restaurants and fast-food eateries.

126

Fried Foods Cause Irreversible Mutations in Our Cells

Frying any kind of food in the oils and fats just discussed makes it hazardous, even if the food itself is not a promoter of free radicals. For instance, potatoes are a health-enhancing plant food. But when fried, they become a risk factor for cancer or heart disease. Vegetables like broccoli, carrots, eggplant or spinach—all virtually fat-free—act like sponges when fried in oils or fats that promote free radicals. In the frying pan, a single serving typically sops up 3 teaspoons of oil, equivalent to 15 grams of fat. Yet if stir-fried, sauteed in nonstick spray or steamed, these vegetables stay almost fat-free.

Other recent tests at Texas Tech University Health Sciences Center discovered that frying (or even broiling) any flesh food to the well-done stage produced carcinogens called *heterocyclic amines.* This was true also of fish and poultry.

Besides health-destroying fats, the foods that promote free radicals contain excessive amounts of protein as well as potentially harmful remnants of growth hormones and antibiotics. Except for calcium in dairy products, these foods are really a nutritional wasteland. More fat and protein are the last nutrients most Americans need. And while these foods may contain a few vitamins and minerals, almost all these nutrients are available in less-risky foods that grow on plants.

Why We Should Avoid Foods That Promote Free Radicals

The real problem with foods that promote free radicals is that none contain any appreciable fiber. Nor do they contain

127

any phytomins, the recently discovered micronutrients that prevent cancer and heart disease.

Called phytomins because they exist only in plant foods, these wonder nutrients are described in full in IB #4. Virtually all fruits, vegetables, whole grains, legumes and other foods that grow on plants are rich, first, in antioxidants that neutralize and mop up free radicals. And second, in a series of powerful anticarcinogens, each capable of preventing or retarding cancer or even slowing or blocking further growth of a small cancerous tumor.

Don't look for any of these incredible nutrients in any food of animal origin, including dairy products and eggs, or in any of the oils and fats that promote free radicals.

Sobering Studies Reveal Why Our Immune Systems Are Suppressed

Cancer, largely responsible for overloading and therefore weakening our immune systems, is rapidly overtaking heart disease as the leading cause of death in America. According to the American Cancer Society, almost one-third of all cancers are caused by dietary factors. And just about all of these factors involve foods that promote free radicals.

For example, the latest American Cancer Society guidelines recommend cutting out all red meat, not merely high-fat meat. They link meat consumption to cancers of the colon, prostate, rectum and endometrium.

Similar findings turned up in the huge and ongoing Nurses' Health Study. All indications showed that a high intake of saturated fat increases bile production by the liver, and a breakdown of this bile releases free radicals that cause colon tumors. Beef, lamb and pork were most strongly linked to colon cancer, especially in women who ate these meats as a main course several times a week. Researchers concluded that eating just one-third of an ounce of saturated fat (10 grams) daily can put a person at risk for colon cancer. Other studies have also found that consuming 10 grams of saturated fat per day significantly increased the risk for breast cancer.

Additional confirmation comes from a study of almost 50,000 male health professionals reported in the 1993 *Journal of the National Cancer Society* (85: 15/1), which found that men who eat meat four to five times a week as a main dish have four times more risk of colon cancer as men who eat meat less than once a month. The same study also concluded that heavy meat-eaters were twice as likely to get prostate cancer—even if the meat was lean.

I could go on and on reporting similar findings by one major study after another. A study from Uruguay, for example, reports that women who ate the most meat had more than three times the risk of breast cancer as women who ate the least meat. Another study by Brian Chu, Ph.D. at the University of Iowa found that women who ate four hamburgers or more per month had almost twice the risk of developing non-Hodgkin's lymphoma (a cancer of the lymph system) as women who ate fewer hamburgers.

Literally scores of large studies from around the world have each implicated meat and fat as a prime cause of most cancers. And anyone who has read this book this far will understand the plain fact that indirectly meat and fat are also major suppressors of our immune systems.

But this Immune Booster has covered only a single way in which foods that promote free radicals suppress our immunity. Immune Boosters #5 and #6 reveal how a fat-laden diet sends our BMI soaring and how being overweight has a devastating effect on immuno-competence.

129

IMMUNE BOOSTER #4: The One Diet That Does It All

Imagine a diet that could prevent up to 75 percent or more of heart disease and cancer and nearly all the other diseases that afflict and kill older Americans, that could restore most peoples' weight to normal, that could slow the aging process and that could give us the immunity and the arteries, heart, lungs and digestion of the average person half our age. And in the process, it can also help supercharge our immunity.

What's the catch? you may ask. Surely, if this were true, it would be the greatest health discovery in history. It would prevent most of modern humanity's worst diseases. It would eliminate a huge amount of pain and suffering. It would save billions in medical costs. And everyone would be eating these foods.

That's what any logical-thinking person might expect. But despite wide coverage in the media, news of this super-healthy diet has been largely ignored and people are continuing to eat almost exactly as they did before.

What is this amazing new diet? First, although I talk about "diet" here, it's not really a diet, but an entirely new way of looking at food that ensures you will make only wise food choices. To get started, you need take only two simple steps.

Step 1. Cut back or, if possible, eliminate from your diet all of the foods listed in IB #3 that promote free radicals.

Step 2. Replace these health-robbing foods with health-building foods that grow on plants and that abound in fiber, antioxidants and anticarcinogens.

130

All the health-building foods we should eat more of grow on plants. You'll find most of them listed below.

THE FOODS THAT SUPERCHARGE OUR IMMUNE SYSTEM

By Defending Us Against Cancer, Obesity and Premature Aging

Vegetables: artichokes, asparagus, beets, black beans, black-eyed peas, bok choy, broccoli, brussels sprouts, cabbage, carrots, cauliflower, celery, chard, chives, collard greens, cucumber, dried beans, eggplant, endive, garbanzos, garlic, green beans, green leafy vegetables, green and red peppers, kale, kidney beans, kohlrabi, leeks, lentils, lettuce (except iceberg), lima beans, mustard greens, okra, onions, parsnips, peas, potatoes, roasted soybeans, rutabagas, scallions, shallots, soybeans, spinach, squash, sweet potatoes, Swiss chard, tomatoes and tomato sauce, turnips, turnip greens and watercress.

Fruits: apricots (fresh or dried), avocadoes, bananas, berries, blackberries, cantaloupe, citrus, cranberries, figs, grapes, grapefruit, guavas, kiwi fruit, mangoes, melons, oranges, papaya, peaches, pears, persimmons, pineapples, plums, prunes, raisins, strawberries, tangerines and watermelons.

Whole Grains: barley, brown rice, buckwheat, corn, kasha, oats and oatmeal, popcorn (air popped and plain), rye, wheat bran, products made of 100 percent whole wheat and most other whole grain products.

131

Other Healthful Foods Derived from Plants: flaxseed, miso, all types of nuts, soy milk, soy protein, sunflower and other seeds, tea (black, green or oolong), tempeh and tofu.

Nature's Own Anticancer Nutrition Plan

All these foods grow on, or are derived, from plants. A diet of these foods is called a *plant-based diet*. This is in contrast to the earlier term *vegetarian*, which nowadays implies abstaining only from meat. A plant-based diet also excludes all of the foods that promote free radicals (listed in IB# 3) and all of the foods that promote weight gain (listed in IB# 6).

When it comes to protecting your immunity, most foods fall into one of two classes.

"Bad guy" foods that promote free radicals, are primarily of animal origin or are high in saturated or polyunsaturated fats or trans-fatty acids.

"Good guy" foods, consisting of fruits, vegetables, whole grains, legumes, nuts and seeds that all grow on plants, are low in fat and rarely promote free radicals. These foods are high in fiber and they abound in phytomins (antioxidants and anticarcinogens) as well as in most vitamins and minerals.

'Neutral" foods include canola, flaxseed and olive oils: these primarily monounsaturated oils produce few free radicals. If you must use fats or oils, these are far preferable to those listed in IB #3. (However, they still consist 100 percent of fat. And they can make you overweight, which appears to be a risk factor for hormone-related cancers.)

132

Other neutral foods are plain nonfat dairy foods, which also do not appear to promote free radicals, white flour, white bread and sugar—indeed all sweeteners including molasses, honey and high-fructose corn syrup—which may contain a few vitamins and minerals but in reality are little more than empty calories.

The problem with all these neutral foods is that none contain any appreciable fiber or any of the phytomins that protect against cancer and heart disease.

When More Is Better

When we eat foods other than nonfat dairy and "good guy" foods, we create a situation known as *negative attrition.* That means the more "bad guy" and neutral foods we consume, the less room we have in our stomachs for the "good guy" foods that grow on plants. And though we know that more is not always better, when it comes to eating plant-based foods, the more we eat the healthier we, and our immune systems, become.

Phytomins give plants their color, flavor and odor. Several hundred may exist in a single plant food, and hundreds of phytomins work together as a team to destroy free radicals and prevent the formation of cancer cells. More than 500 different varieties have already been analyzed, and scientists have identified 14 different classes of phytomins in plant-based foods.

While most evidence comes from lab and animal studies and is still considered preliminary, it is already so overwhelming that human studies are only expected to confirm what has already been discovered.

133

Why Antioxidants Exist Primarily in Plant-Based
Foods

The function of plants is to oxidize carbon into carbohydrates using solar energy. In doing so, plants release huge amounts of oxygen and free radicals. Despite all this, plants are virtually immune to free radical damage.

The explanation? Plants also produce enormous quantities of antioxidants that sop up and snuff out their free radicals. When we eat an abundance of plant-based foods, we absorb such generous amounts of antioxidants that free radical damage in our bodies is slowed to a crawl.

When we eat phytomins in plants, we are actually eating the plant's immune system. Just about all plants that grow in sunlight contain hundreds of different phytomins. Many of these, such as flavonoids, glutathione and polyphenols, are both antioxidants *and* anticarcinogens. Hundreds of others are powerful anticarcinogens and they work in a variety of ways to prevent cancer. Some also block the growth of cancer and small tumors. Thus the more plant foods we eat, the richer our diet is in fiber and phytomins and the lower our risk of forming cancer cells.

Why Are Plant Foods So Essential?

During millions of years of human evolution, the metabolism of our ancestors came to depend on the plant foods they gathered. These foods provided vital chemicals that our bodies cannot make and that are totally lacking in flesh foods, eggs and dairy products.

Today, we know these vital chemicals as phytomins and we need them every bit as much as our ancestors did. Since they create conditions unfavorable to tumor formation in

134

skin cells that line our inner organs, many phytomins are just as essential as vitamins and minerals—and probably more so. It is in cells deep within the body—in the lining of the bladder, cervix, colon, esophagus, larynx, lung, pancreas, stomach and throat—that many cancers begin.

Including a moderate amount of phytomins in our diet— by eating, say, nine servings of fruits and vegetables and eight or more servings of whole grains each day—is estimated to cut the risk of most cancers by close to 50 percent. But a number of population studies, including the famous China Health Study, have suggested that eating a diet composed exclusively of plant foods could reduce cancer risk by 50 to 90 percent. Supporting this view is the fact that more than 150 major studies have shown that a person who eats an abundance of plant foods every day has less than half the risk of cancer, diabetes or heart disease as the general population.

When broken down, these studies revealed that people who eat two or more servings of fruits and vegetables per day are 40 percent more likely to get cancer of the colon, esophagus, lung and stomach than people who eat five or more servings. This gave rise to the "Five-a-Day" slogan you may see in supermarket produce departments. It's sound advice. But it fails to go far enough. On its Food Pyramid, the USDA recommends up to nine servings of fruits and vegetables per day and up to eleven servings of whole grains (breads, cereals, pasta and rice).

If that sounds like a lot it's because, according to the *American Journal of Public Health*, only 20 percent of adults actually consume five servings each day. The average American eats only 3.5 servings of fruits and vegetables and a mere two tablespoons of beans. On any given day, half of all Americans eat no fruit and that includes children.

Many authors of these studies have suggested that failure

135

to consume sufficient fruits, vegetables, whole grains and other plant foods is responsible for most of the chronic diseases that afflict Western nations.

We all know that plant foods are rich in fiber, vitamins and minerals. But our need for phytomins goes far beyond these well-known nutrients. Here, to introduce these nutritional "good guys," is a detailed breakdown of the leading phytomins and how each one can help beat cancer up front before it can overburden the immune system.

Carotenoids

More than 600 different carotenoids found in yellow, orange and dark green fruits and vegetables work together in complexes to destroy free radicals. Some work best as antioxidants to prevent cancer; others function best to prevent eye and heart diseases caused by free radicals. However, by eating a variety of fruits and vegetables, you can obtain complete antioxidant coverage against most diseases caused by free radicals.

Five principal carotenoid groups exist: alpha-carotene, beta-carotene, beta cryptoxanthin, lutein and lycopene. (We will only discuss the two major ones—beta-carotene and lycopene—here.)

Beta-Carotene

Beta-carotene was one of the first antioxidants to be discovered, and supplements containing this single nutrient were extensively tested for their effectiveness in preventing cancer and heart disease. In many cases, the results were disappointing. Meanwhile, other studies done on foods known to contain beta-carotene, such as carrots, winter squash and yams, proved highly successful.

For example, a National Cancer Institute study in 1986 found that male smokers who ate only half a cup of yams, sweet potatoes or winter squash every day cut their risk of lung cancer in half. At the time, researchers were unaware that these vegetables contained not one or two groups of carotenes but all five. Additionally, each was packed with hundreds of other disease-fighting compounds.

It was these hundreds of carotenoids and other phytomins working together, not merely the beta-carotene category alone, that slashed the risk of lung and other cancers. In fact, many researchers now suspect that beta-carotene is merely a marker for other, far more effective anticarcinogens that exist in the same plant foods as beta-carotene. Foods with a high beta-carotene content have been found to lower risk of lung and possibly bladder, colon, esophagus, larynx, mouth, pancreas, stomach and throat cancers.

Lycopene

In 1996, a major study demonstrated that the carotene lycopene dramatically slowed the onset and growth of colon and prostate cancers. Men who ate 10 or more servings of tomato products each week had significantly lower rates of both cancers. Based on the number of micrograms of lycopene per 100 grams of food, the best lycopene sources are:

Tomato sauce, canned	6,500	Tomato, raw	3,100
Watermelon, raw	4,100	Pink grapefruit, raw	3,362

Pound for pound, sun-dried tomatoes appear to be 17 times as rich in micronutrients as fresh tomatoes. And vine-ripened

137

fresh tomatoes are also far superior to the typical supermarket tomato which is picked green and ripened with ethylene gas. In fact, most commercial tomatoes are tasteless and have a lower content of vitamins, antioxidants and phytomins. You can identify a vine-ripened tomato because it smells like a tomato. Gassed tomatoes are odorless. For this reason, tomato sauce or canned tomatoes may contain more lycopene.

Sulphur Compounds

Chives, garlic, leeks, onions, scallions and shallots all contain highly active sulphur compounds believed to help immobilize cancer of the colon, liver, lung and stomach. An invitro study at New York's Memorial-Sloan Kettering Cancer Center a few years ago found that four compounds in garlic helped retard initiation of breast cells with cancer by transforming estrogen into noncarcinogenic forms.

Numerous studies have identified anticarcinogenic phytomins in garlic. Animal studies at Penn State University made in the early 1990s indicated that garlic could inhibit the rate of breast cancer growth by 70 percent. Another animal study by Benjamin Lau, M.D. at Loma Linda University School of Medicine in California found that compounds in garlic may stimulate macrophages, T4 and NK cells to migrate to a cancer site. Tests were made on a variety of cancer sites and garlic appeared to inhibit the entire cancer process, even in small tumors.

Another study, conducted at Johns Hopkins School of Medicine on 41,837 women over a 5-year period, discovered that women who ate garlic regularly had a 50 percent lower risk of colon cancer. Still another study by Dr. B. Torok at the University of Tubingen in Germany found that antioxidants in garlic zapped free radicals released by cigarette smoke.

Dialkyl sulphides, the compound that gives garlic its odor, have been observed to slow the growth of cancer of the colon, esophagus and stomach in lab animals. Dialkyl sulphides have also blocked cholesterol synthesis by the liver in response to a high-fat diet.

It is highly probable that the entire allium (onion) family contains approximately the same phytomins as garlic. For instance, one large study in the Netherlands followed 121,000 men and women aged 55 to 69. After 10 years, results showed that those who consumed at least half of one medium-sized onion per day had the lowest incidence of stomach cancer.

The phytomins in garlic may also work topically. One study made at New York University Medical Center during the 1980s showed that when garlic oil was applied to skin tumors, it slowed the growth of skin cancer. In the same study, test animals given garlic developed only one-fourth as many colon tumors as those fed a straight diet of grain.

While allium vegetables have failed to prevent breast cancer, many nutritionists believe that garlic and other onion family foods should be part of any anticancer diet. It's interesting to note that cooking doesn't seem to inhibit the action of allium vegetables.

It's best to eat four cloves of garlic daily as a food seasoning. To avoid having your breath smell of garlic, try garlic powder, available in most supermarkets. It's cheaper than garlic capsules and contains more nutrients. Many nutritionists suspect that odor-free garlic supplements contain fewer nutrients.

Ellagic Acid

This important antioxidant is believed to help protect the DNA of body cells by blocking penetration of free radicals through cell walls. Apples, blackberries, cranberries, grapes, raspberries and strawberries are all rich in ellagic acid. Since ellagic acid is rarely damaged by cooking, freezing or preserving, jams, juices and frozen berries are often excellent sources.

Flavonoids

Flavonoids are antioxidants. They also appear to reduce the rate of cancer metastases by blocking cancer-promoting enzymes from binding on to receptors in healthy cells.

For more than 25 years, 12 university medical schools in seven countries have followed the diets of 5,000 people. Those consuming the most flavonoids have consistently developed less cancer and heart disease than those eating the least. Foods rich in flavonoids are apples, berries, broccoli, carrots, grapes, onions, peppers and tomatoes. Regular consumption of black, green or oolong tea has also been linked to reduced risk of cancer of the esophagus, lung, pancreas, rectum, skin and stomach. Each of these teas has a high flavonoid content.

Studies on primates have also found that a flavonoid-rich diet helps prevent cholesterol deposits from forming in coronary arteries. It also prevents the blood clots that trigger most heart attacks and strokes.

Further confirmation emerged in 1996 when an in-vitro study at the Center for Human Nutrition at the University of Western Ontario found that two flavonoids in tangerines

140

helped retard the growth of breast cancer cells. Known as tangeretin and nobiletin, these phytomins are to be tested next on animals, then on humans.

Many women health professionals aren't waiting for test results. They're already eating at least one tangerine daily as insurance against developing breast cancer. Incidentally, the same study discovered that flavonoids in grapefruit juice were almost as effective.

Indoles

Indoles are a class of nitrogen compounds that inhibit hormone-dependent cancers by inactivating estrogen in the body. Three different types of indoles exist and all are potent cancer fighters.

The *Indole-3-Carbinol (I3C)* type abounds in cruciferous vegetables such as bok choy, broccoli, brussels sprouts, cabbage, cauliflower, collards, kale, kohlrabi, mustard greens, rutabagas, turnips, turnip greens and watercress. (Since overcooking damages most indoles, these foods are best eaten raw, lightly steamed or cooked and still crunchy.)

Animal studies have shown that I3C indoles appear to prevent carcinogens from activating initiated cancer cells. For instance, during a 1991 study at the Foundation for Preventive Oncology, New York, researchers concluded that I3C blocked the chemical process that leads to breast cancer. While clinical studies have yet to be done, surveys of people who eat liberal amounts of cruciferous vegetables show a 50 percent lower incidence of cancers of the breast, colon and rectum and a significant reduction in other types of cancer.

Lignans are another type of indole found in soybeans and all soy-based products and in barley, flaxseed, wheat and other whole grains. Lignans are believed to inhibit activation of initiated cancer cells. Surveys of Hispanics and American Indians, who eat more grains, suggest that lignans may be responsible for their lower incidence of breast and colon cancer. Other research has indicated that lignans may help subdue the autoimmune response that causes the immune system to attack the self.

Flaxseed contains lignan precursors which are transformed in the body, into low-level estrogens that behave like isoflavones (see below). In animal studies, lignan precursors in flaxseed have prevented formation of breast cancer tumors and slowed the growth of small tumors already in place. Flaxseed is also rich in alpha linoleic fatty acid which is believed to slow the growth of breast cancer tumors.

Many nutritionists recommend eating one serving (2.5 grams) of flaxseed each day but only a small amount is needed). (2.5 grams is just one-tenth of an ounce,). Half a teaspoon of flaxseed equals about 2.5 grams. For best results, eat the seeds, not the oil. Because ground flaxseed quickly becomes rancid, we grind whole flaxseed in a pestel and mortar just prior to use. Some people sprinkle it on their breakfast cereal, or they dissolve it in juice. Others make muffins that contain approximately 2.5 grams of flaxseed each.

Dithiolthiones, another type of indole, stimulates the release of glutathione, an important cancer fighter reviewed below.

Glutathione

One of the most powerful anticarcinogens ever found in plant foods, glutathione is synthesized in the body from amino acids in plant foods. But anyone who consumes fewer than nine servings of fruits and vegetables daily may have a deficiency. For example, glutathione levels in people over 60 tend to average 17 percent lower than in people under 40. Most of us can use all the glutathione we can get.

Lab tests found that this potent anticancer compound enhances production of enzymes that neutralize free radicals and sweep carcinogens out of the body before either can penetrate body cells.

In one study, when glutathione was fed to cancer prone hamsters, those given glutathione grew tumors only one-tenth as large as hamsters that did not receive glutathione. In other animal studies, glutathione prevented diabetes and obesity in mice genetically prone to those diseases.

Foods rich in glutathione include arugula, asparagus, avocadoes, broccoli, cabbage, cantaloupe, citrus fruits and juices, kale, mustard greens, okra, peaches, strawberries, tomatoes, watercress, watermelons and winter squash. Glutathione is best absorbed when plant foods are eaten raw.

Isoflavones

Why do Americans have 8.7 times more breast cancer and 30 times more prostate cancer than most people in Asia who still eat a traditional soy-rich diet? The answer, researchers discovered, is because Koreans, Vietnamese and others consume an average of 60 grams (2 ounces) of soy products each day, while most Americans eat none.

Soy products are rich in isoflavones, a class of phytomins that contain plant estrogens. Though relatively weak, these phytoestrogens interact with estrogens in the bodies of both women and men. They then intervene in the cancer process on three different levels.

143

First, isoflavones appear to inhibit estrogen-promoted cancers such as cancer of the breast and prostate. They do so by binding with the same receptors in breast and prostate cells used by body estrogens. By occupying all estrogen receptors, isoflavones prevent body estrogen from binding on to these receptors and promoting cancer.

Second, certain isoflavones appear to prevent angiogenesis. This virtually halts the growth of small, malignant tumors.

Third, a diet high in isoflavones may also lengthen the menstrual cycle by roughly 2.5 days. When this happens, less body estrogen is secreted with each ovulation. In turn, this reduces the rate of cell division in the breast, thus minimizing the chances of cell mutations.

Genistein: Soy Against Cancer

Genistein and daidzen are the two most common isoflavones. Since they are found together and work as a team, only genistein is mentioned here.

Though no human studies have been completed to date, genistein has retarded growth of prostate tumors in mice, even when the mice were given a high-fat diet. In one study at the University of Tennessee, researchers put genistein into a petri dish with prostate cancer cells. Within a day, the isoflavones had halted cancer cell activity. In lab studies, genistein has consistently retarded the division of breast cancer cells while permitting normal cells to continue growing.

Genistein also appears to control the surges of estrogen that appear during the menstrual cycle and that may well be a partial cause of breast cancer. In all animal studies, in fact, isoflavones have provided significant protection from tumor formation, including cancer of the colon, esophagus, liver and lung. Additionally, soy products (in which isofla-vones abound) have lowered elevated cholesterol in men at risk for heart disease and inhibited further blockage of the coronary arteries. These studies strongly suggest that gen-istein blocks angiogenesis

Other Isoflavones

Soy products also contain four other isoflavones that help fight cancer:

Caffeic acid helps the body sweep out carcinogens by mak-ing them soluble in water.

Ferulic acid prevents nitrates in sausage and luncheon meats from being transformed into nitrosamines, which are potent carcinogens.

Photosterols help prevent colon cancer by blocking repro-duction of activated cancer cells in the large intestine.

Saponins, by blocking DNA division in cancer cells, pre-vent activated cells from multiplying. Saponins may also lower elevated blood cholesterol levels. They are found in many herbs and vegetables.

The average Asian woman eating a traditional diet con-sumes 50 mg of isoflavones daily, primarily from soy prod-ucts. To ensure a similar intake, you should include at least one serving of soy-based foods per day.

The best sources are soybeans, both raw and roasted, tofu, soy milk, flour or protein isolate. Since tofu is quite high in fat and calories, 1 percent lowfat tofu is the best choice. Tofu can be cut or crumbled into small pieces and used in many foods and salads. Defatted soy flour can also be used in any baked goods recipe by replacing one-fourth of the wheat flour. Plain soy milk can also be used for baking. And rehydrated textured vegetable protein (also called *soy protein isolate*) makes an excellent substitute for ground meat.

Besides being packed with isoflavones, most soy products are also rich sources of other nutrients. For example, 4 tablespoons of roasted soybeans contain 22 percent of the RDA for folic acid, 14 percent of the RDA for zinc, 25 percent of the RDA for magnesium and lots of fiber. Other foods that contain appreciable amounts of isoflavones are black-eyed peas, fava beans, garbanzos, kidney beans, lentils, lima beans and most other dried beans, peas and seeds.

However, it's important to note that soy sauce, soybean oil, soy formulas or soy-based drinks all have a low isoflavone content.

Isothiocyanates

This class of phytomins, which includes sulforaphane, is believed to stimulate the mobilization of enzymes known to deactivate cancer cells. Experiments with rats showed that foods high in isothiocyanates slowed breast cancer growth. Similar animal studies have strongly suggested that isothiocyanates weaken the carcinogenic effects of cigarette smoke and may even inhibit lung cancer due to cigarette smoking. Isothiocyanates are abundant in all cruciferous vegetables and also in mustard greens and horseradish.

Protease Inhibitors

Besides isoflavones, soy-based foods abound in phytomins called *protease inhibitors*. Doctors are now using very powerful protease inhibitors produced by pharmaceutical companies to treat AIDS, with dramatic life-prolonging results.

In animal studies, protease inhibitors from soybeans suppressed cancer formation in a number of sites. Experiments have shown that this class of phytomins interferes with the secretion of enzymes by cancer cells that are essential for tumor formation and growth.

Other Phytomins

Though few studies have yet been completed, preliminary indications reveal that other classes of phytomins found only in plant foods are also powerful cancer fighters, including:

Anthocyanins found in Concord grapes, eggplant, radishes and red cabbage.

Capsaicin found in hot peppers.

Coumarins found in citrus fruits, cucumber, parsley, parsnips and tomatoes.

Glucarates found in citrus fruits, cruciferous vegetables, eggplant, peppers, tomatoes and whole grains.

Monoterpenes found in a wide variety of vegetables and in citrus fruits; also in fennel and caraway seeds.

Phenolic acid and triterpines both found in many vegetables, citrus fruits and whole grains.

Phthalides and Polyacetylenes both found in carrots, celery, fennel, parsley and parsnips.

Phytates found in soy products and whole grains.

S-allycysteine found in allium vegetables.

147

Another Cancer-Fighting Nutrient in "Good Guy" Foods

Irrefutable evidence exists that foods high in fiber significantly cut cancer and heart disease risk. Fiber also lowers the body's store of fat and helps restore BMI to normal (25 or less; see IB #5). Both cancer and being overweight cause immuno-suppression.

A dozen major studies, including the China Health Study, have clearly indicated that people who eat more fiber have a much lower risk of cancer mortality. For instance, high estrogen levels are regarded as a marker for increased breast cancer risk. But fiber reduces this risk by binding with natural hormones in the body and speeding their elimination. This ability was indicated recently during a small study of 12 women at UCLA School of Medicine. When the 12 were given a high-fiber diet, their overall estrogen level dropped by 30 percent.

Supporting this conclusion were findings from a study in Finland; women who consumed 30 grams of fiber daily had only half the breast cancer of women who consumed only 14 grams. Another European study found that consuming 30 grams of fiber daily cut the production of women's estrogen levels by one-fifth.

A high-fiber intake also prevents colon cancer by speeding up the digestion process so that carcinogenic food wastes do not linger in the colon. In one study in which people prone to colon cancer ate a high-fiber diet, production of cancer-causing bile acids fell by more than half.

In recent years, other research has proved that eating high-fiber foods is an essential step in restoring your weight (or BMI) to normal. It's not merely a matter of switching from high-fat to low-fat foods, researchers found. Replacing high-fat cookies with low-fat cookies, for instances, has little effect. To really start your weight sliding, you need to switch from high-fat cookies to "good guy" foods, especially such high-fiber champions as barley, beans, prunes or raisin bran cereal. The same studies also discovered that, unsurprisingly, most overweight women have a 30 percent deficiency in fiber intake.

Test Yourself to See If You Are Getting Sufficient Fiber

If your stools are hard or dark, or if you don't move your bowels at least once a day, it could indicate a possible deficiency of dietary fiber. Being constipated, even occasionally, is another indication that you may need additional fiber.

For most people, breakfast is the most fiber-rich meal of the day. So if you skip breakfast, or just grab a doughnut, you could be seriously deficient in fiber. By contrast, if your stools are soft and bulky and pass easily, you are probably getting sufficient fiber, especially if your foods are all from the "good guy" category.

For anyone eating a diet high in plant-based foods, bowel transit time averages only 18 to 24 hours. You can check your personal transit time like this: Eat a small serving of whole kernel corn with a meal. Then eat no more corn until the kernels appear in your stool. The time that elapses between eating the corn and seeing it in your stool is your personal transit time.

Anyone who eats a lot of "bad guy" foods (meat, fat, poultry or eggs) may carry the residue of 8 to 11 meals in their colon and have a typical bowel transit time of 3

149

to 4 days. Lack of fiber can turn the colon into a huge holding tank, allowing carcinogens to form and cause colorectal cancer.

How Much Fiber Do We Need to Keep Cancer and Obesity at Bay?

The National Cancer Institute has recommended a daily fiber intake of 20 to 30 grams. But many experts believe that 35 grams would be better, with 10 grams from soluble fiber and 25 grams from insoluble fiber. When you consider that the average American consumes only 10.5 grams per day, it's little wonder that one person in every three develops cancer *and* is seriously overweight.

Everyone knows you can put fiber into "bad guy" foods by adding a few tablespoons of bran. But brans contain just one type of fiber. To prevent the onset of cancer and to normalize weight, we need both soluble and insoluble fiber.

Soluble fiber binds with bile acids and hormones and excretes them from the body. When eaten, it creates a feeling of fullness and satiety that discourages most people from overeating. The best sources of soluble fliber are cooked dried beans, oatmeal and many fruits and vegetables.

Insoluble fiber creates large, bulky stools that sweep through the intestines like a cleansing broom, excreting food wastes at three to four times the speed of "bad guy" foods. In doing so, insoluble fiber carries away many of the hormones and carcinogens that appear to cause breast, colon, colorectal and prostate cancer.

150

For best results, we should consume 10 to 25 grams of insoluble fiber per day. Most plant foods are rich in insoluble fiber, but the best sources are the bran in wheat and oats products, lentils, beans and brown rice. For instance, 1 ounce of wheat or oat bran contains 12 grams of insoluble fiber.

Pack Your Meals With Fiber

The best way to obtain an abundance of both soluble and insoluble fiber is to eat plenty of "good guy" foods, that is, fruits, vegetables, whole grains, legumes, nuts and seeds. To consume 30 grams of fiber daily, we need to eat five to nine servings of fruits and vegetables, five or more servings of whole (unrefined) grains, one serving of a high-fiber cereal like raisin bran and one serving of dried beans, especially soybeans.

Refined wheat products like white bread and flour—anything made with white flour—are poor fiber sources, as are most supermarket breads, except those marked "100 percent whole wheat."

"Good guy" foods with the highest overall fiber content are prunes, barley, black beans, raisin bran cereal, broccoli, apples, brown rice, bran (corn, oats, rice, wheat), brussels sprouts, carrots, cooked lentils and dried beans, cooked grains (buckwheat, corn, kasha, millet, oats, rye, wheat), figs, leeks, onions, peas, plums, baked white potatoes and sweet potatoes. One tip: Not all fiber is in the skin.

THREE WAYS TO HELP PHYTOMINS PROTECT YOUR IMMUNITY

Phytomins can help defend your immunity in three important ways.

Rely Only on Plant Foods for Phytomins

Until recently, it was thought that a single vitamin or mineral, acting as an antioxidant, could prevent cancer or heart disease. Studies show that vitamins C, E, cysteine, folic acid, selenium and zinc may all have worthwhile antioxidant or anticarcinogenic properties. Yet their effect is limited compared with that of the hundreds of micronutrients found in a single plant food. For instance, most single nutrient antioxidants are site-specific, meaning they work on only one type of cancer in one single body location.

By comparison, phytomins can intervene in the cancer process on almost every level. Researchers describe phytomins as possessing anticarcinogenic and antimutational properties, meaning they fight cancer in a variety of ways. For example, they may block initiation and activation of cancer by neutralizing free radicals. Others boost the activity of enzymes that can detoxify carcinogens. Some produce hormones that neutralize hormones in the body that promote hormone-related cancers. Yet others can block angiogenesis in small tumors. And still others are able to inhibit reactive carcinogens.

Findings show that it is the variety and assortment of phytomins working together that prevent cancer, not merely a few single nutrients in an extract or supplement. Each phytomin group supports and enhances the benefits of every other phytomin. Therefore we need to maintain the whole spectrum of phytomins in our bodies.

I'm not trying to dissuade you from taking vitamin or mineral supplements. IB #2 suggests a number of vitamins and minerals that may help boost your immunity. But researchers have learned that we also need to eat a variety of "good guy" foods, each of which contains a complex assortment of weak antioxidents and anticarcinogens. When eaten together, these micronutrients provide powerful resistance to cancer formation.

This fact is currently being confirmed by the Women's Healthy Eating and Living Trial, a study based on a diet high in plant foods and fiber and low in fat. One 7-year study of 34,000 postmenopausal women, completed at the University of Minnesota and released in 1996, has already revealed that by eating foods rich in vitamin E, particularly nuts and seeds, participants obtained better protection against heart disease than a control group taking vitamin E alone. Another test showed that eating a whole orange supplies several times more phytomins than drinking a comparable amount of orange juice, though the juice has a higher vitamin C content.

In conclusion, phytomins are the most exciting disease-fighting nutrients to have been discovered in recent times. But they cannot be found in a bottle or pill. To benefit from their discovery, we have to eat an abundance of "good guy" foods—real fruits and vegetables and other foods that grow on plants—instead of the "bad guy" foods that tear down our bodies and weaken our immunity.

Eat a Balanced Diet of "Good Guy" Foods

A recent Harvard School of Public Health study on Greek women with breast cancer showed that vegetables provided slightly greater cancer protection than fruits. This confirms the old rule that we should eat two servings of vegetables for every one of fruit. Additionally, we need whole grains, legumes and some nuts and seeds in our diet.

For most of us, a mix of five servings of vegetables and four of fruit each day plus 6 to 11 servings of whole grain breads or cereals, one or more servings of legumes and a few nuts and seeds is an ideal target to shoot for. As we become accustomed to eating these "good guy" foods, we can up the amounts of vegetables and fruits.

These amounts are not nearly as large as you probably think. For most cooked foods, one serving equals only half a cupful. For smaller fruits like apples, citrus and bananas, one serving equals one whole fruit. One slice of bread equals one serving, as does a comparable weight and volume of other whole grain cereals. One serving of bulky, chopped raw vegetables like lettuce usually equals one cupful.

For most people, these are quite small amounts. But put together, they provide us with one giant anticancer cocktail that supercharges our bodies with disease-fighting phytomins.

"Good Guy" Foods Provide Gourmet Meals and New Eating Adventures

To maximize fiber and phytomin absorption, just about all fruits and salad-type vegetables are best eaten raw. For tubers, grains and legumes, microwaving, followed by steaming or baking, causes the least nutrient loss.

154

Eating "good guy" foods doesn't have to be bland or unexciting. Plant-based foods supply a splendid opportunity to discover a whole new world of exciting taste treats and culinary adventures. As I wrote in my earlier book, *Eighteen Natural Ways to Lower Your Cholesterol*:

> *Far from tasting bland or drab, plant-based recipes can provide peak experiences in cooking taste and enjoyment. You don't have to live on sprouts and carrots. All the rich, subtle flavors and pungent seasonings of exotic Third World countries are yours to enjoy.*
>
> *From countries where the average cholesterol level is far lower than ours come hundreds of exciting, heart-healthy recipes. To sample the pastas of Italy, the curries of South India or the bouillabaisse of Provence will quickly convince you that "gourmet cooking" is compatible with low cholesterol. From the great culinary traditions of China, Japan and India, you can draw on dozens of tasty grain-based dishes, virtually every one free of saturated fat and cholesterol.*
>
> *In Mediterreanean countries, where olive oil adds luster to every food, people traditionally eat only small, lean portions of meat and few, if any, dairy foods.*

Other ways to spice up your cooking include preparing rich stews and soups using a vegetable broth of sauteed onions, peppers and mushrooms. Try whole grain pasta, vegetable chili or lentil soup with a heavy serving of tomato paste or sauce. Use mushrooms in place of meat. For a princely salad, mix grilled mushrooms with salad greens. Enliven the taste of tempeh or tofu by crumbling it into casseroles, chilis or pasta sauces. Or broil, grill or sautee marinated tempeh or tofu.

155

If you need a meat substitute, try meatless burgers or weiners or patties made with grains, seeds or soy.

Plant foods are best eaten fresh. They can lose phytomins when stored in a refrigerator or on shelves. When fresh foods are unavailable, frozen or canned vegetables are alternate sources of phytomins. A good rule is that the fresher a fruit or vegetable, the higher its nutrient value. For this reason, it's best to avoid pre-cut fruits like melons or on-sale vegetables, though firm bananas speckled with brown spots are often a good buy when offered at half price.

Yogurt to the Rescue

Plain nonfat yogurt is a healthful substitute for cream or salad dressings. Although findings are preliminary, one study at Long Island Jewish Medical Center, New York, demonstrated that the incidence of chronic yeast infection fell 66 percent when women ate a cup of yogurt containing live bacteria each day for six months. Another small study at Tufts University involved women over 60 who were deficient in a stomach acid that helps prevent colon cancer. When the women ate yogurt containing live bacteria for several weeks, the active cultures in the yogurt replaced the missing stomach acid.

In yet another study at the University of California, people who ate two cups of bacteria-containing yogurt daily for several months produced more gamma-interferon than people in a control group who ate yogurt free of bacteria.

In each of these studies, the active bacterial agent in the yogurt was a live culture of *Lactobacillus acidophilus*. All yogurt containing *L. acidophilus* states the fact on the label. But tests at Tufts University found that the actual acidophilus content varied widely from one brand of yogurt to another and even differed from batch to batch of the same brand.

In addition plain nonfat yogurt is a splendid source of calcium. It can also be eaten by people who are lactose intolerant and unable to eat other dairy products.

An Ice Cream Substitute That KOs Free Radicals

For a wonderfully healthful substitute for ice cream, slice up several ripe fruits such as a banana, kiwi, mango, pear or persimmon; place in a bowl and smother with plain nonfat yogurt. Even teenagers agree that this fruit salad beats the taste of regular ice cream. Besides conventional ice cream contains neither fiber nor phytomins and, excepting calcium, precious little else of any nutritional value but harmful fat and sugar.

From a nutritional viewpoint, it's difficult to eat too many plant foods. Most of us need all the phytomins we can obtain. But it's smart, at first, to ease your way gradually into a plant-based diet. This gives your colon time to adjust to the high-fiber content of plant-based foods. Each week, add one or two new fruits and vegetables while you gradually increase your intake of whole grains and beans.

Some people prefer to make every second meal plant-based while they continue to eat conventional, but less fat-laden, meals in between. Meanwhile, just as gradually, phase out the "bad guy" foods that remain in your diet. Eventually, all your meals can consist of foods that grow on plants.

To help minimize bloating or flatulence, be sure to soak all legumes before cooking and throw away the soaking water. Another good tip is to avoid mixing cabbage-type vege-

157

tables with beans. Don't forget, too, that almost all plant foods are high in fiber and may require more chewing (a factor to consider if you wear dentures). Since fiber sops up water from the intestines, try to drink at least six to eight glasses of water or other nonalcoholic fluids each day.

Follow these guidelines and you should easily make the transition to a plant-based diet in 3 or 4 weeks.

READ THIS BEFORE YOU SWITCH TO A PLANT-BASED DIET

While phytomins in plant foods may help prevent cancer, and even retard or block the growth of small tumors, they are not a *cure* for cancer (nor for AIDS or many other serious diseases). Once cancer symptoms appear, the tumor is usually too large to be blocked by either phytomins or the immune system, and you should seek medical diagnosis and advice. Phytomins are also not a substitute for having periodic medical exams, mammograms or other tests for cancer.

However, with your physician's approval, an abundance of fruits, vegetables, whole grains, legumes, nuts and seeds in the diet may well help prevent a recurrence of cancer that has already been treated.

If you have any degenerative condition which might be adversely affected by adopting a plant-based diet or if you have had surgery on your gastrointestinal tract or have kidney disease, diabetes or any other type of digestive disorder, you should obtain medical clearance before adopting a plant-based diet.

Note that anyone undergoing chemotherapy may also need more dietary fat to keep up his or her weight than is supplied by most plant-based foods.

Conversely, if you're trying to lose excess weight, or if your BMI is over 25, you may wish to cut back on avocadoes, beans, grains, nuts and seeds for a while. Each of these foods contains a certain amount of monounsaturated oils, which, though it rarely promotes free radicals, is still a form of fat that may end up around your middle.

Otherwise, adopting The One Diet That Does It All is an essential step in any program to drop your weight or BMI. It's a given that once you begin eating the "good guy" way you must stay with these healthful foods for the rest of your life. To go back to eating "bad guy" foods is an open invitation to add unwanted weight, bump up your risk of cancer or heart disease and send your immunity skidding.

Don't Be Trapped by the Standard American Diet

Since the health advantages of "good guy" foods are so overwhelming—and you can make scores of tasty grain and vegetable dishes—why doesn't everyone eat The One Diet That Does It All?

The reason is that we live in a huge societal food trap in which everything possible works to dissuade us from eating "good guy" foods. Take the restaurant trap. In any one city, only a handful of restaurants have a salad bar adequate enough to enable us to eat healthfully. Low-fat dishes are not necessarily high in phytomins and fiber. Few fast-food eateries or convenience stores have anything to eat that is not harmful in some way. Yet 57 percent of Americans eat out at least once each day, and many people get half their daily calories at lunch spots and fast-food places that are spawning grounds for free radicals.

Most people are trapped by the eating preferences of the

friends and relatives with whom they eat. At most social events we're expected to break bread with our friends by sharing food they have lovingly prepared—even though it's probably loaded with saturated fat and carcinogens.

Tens of millions of Americans are trapped in a vicious circle of complacency. They've been eating "bad guy" foods for so many years that they're resistant and reluctant to change.

For many of us, the most difficult step in evading the food trap is that the foods most of us love are all "bad guys." Whether they're steak, hamburgers, pizza, fried chicken or shrimp, French fries and pies, cakes, pastries, cookies or ice cream, every last one is a nutritional "bad guy." Eat these foods long enough and you're almost guaranteed a one-way trip to the nearest emergency room. Your immune system may crash and never recover.

Some nutritionists would have you believe there are no "good" or "bad" foods. Yet in the same breath, they advise eating much, much less of what I call "bad guy" foods in this book.

Huge gaps still exist in our knowledge of the chemistry of food and how it affects us in health and disease. But if you're really serious about upgrading your immunity, it should be clear by now that only "good guy" foods can help you do it. And that means you simply cannot afford to remain a victim of the Great American Food Trap.

IMMUNE BOOSTER #5: The 8-Step Weight-Loss and Immune-Boosting Program

---

One American in three is at least 20 pounds overweight, and being this heavy can suppress the immune system in six different ways.

- Excessive body weight has been shown to directly impair the function of killer T-cells and macrophages.
- Excessive body weight significantly increases the risk of cancer of the breast, cervix, endometrium, ovaries and uterus and of the colon, esophagus, gallbladder, kidney, prostate and rectum. Gaining 10 pounds or more in the past few years increases the risk of these cancers even more. As these cancers develop, they can overburden and suppress the immune system.
- Excessive tummy fat, or a potbelly, indicates that a person is overeating in response to stress and releasing stress hormones which directly suppress the immune system.
- Being overweight lowers a person's self-esteem, creating negative emotions which act directly to lower immunocompetence.
- Excessive body weight is closely associated with sedentary living. Lack of exercise drags down every cell in the body, including those of the immune system.

Obviously, excess body weight is toxic to the immune system. Yet in the United States today, the soaring obesity rate has struck every race, sex and age group. Our national obesity epidemic has spawned a multibillion-dollar weight-loss industry that promotes everything from herbs to diet pills, liquid diets and scores of fad diets based on everything from grapefruit to steak, high carbohydrates to low carbohydrates and even diets high in fat and protein.

But dieting doesn't work and never has. After they lose a few pounds, most dieters are unable to stay with their diets. So they go back to eating regular meals and the weight comes piling back. At any one time, 30 million Americans are constantly on some kind of diet, but fewer than 5 percent lose weight permanently.

Poor Body Composition Is What Makes People Overweight

After spending several years studying America's fat problem, researchers at the USDA Jean Mayer Human Nutrition Research Center at Tufts University came up with a new understanding of how we gain weight and why. Whether you're 10 pounds overweight or 100 pounds, being overweight is not the problem, they found. The real problem is having an unhealthy body composition.

Reduced to bare essentials, the human body consists primarily of two components: lean muscle mass and fat. Being overweight, researchers discovered, is caused more by loss of body muscle through lack of exercise than by piling on the fat through overeating.

The explanation is that body muscle is biologically active and burns calories 24 hours a day, even during sleep. Fat, on the other hand, is biologically inactive and burns almost zero calories. Body muscle burns 50 times more calories than body fat. The more muscle we have, the more fat we burn. The more fat we burn, the higher our metabolism. The higher our metabolism, the more slender we become.

Why We Need a High Metabolism

Our metabolism is the number of food calories we need to consume each 24 hours so that our weight remains stable and neither increases nor drops. Under the subhead "Eat Only as Many Calories as Your Body Needs," IB #6 describes an easy way to calculate your personal metabolic rate in just a few minutes. The formula supplies both your resting metabolic rate and your nonresting metabolic rate. Your resting metabolic rate is the number of food calories you consume each day without physical activity. Your nonresting metabolic rate is the number of food calories you consume each day based on your personal level of physical activity.

Our metabolism is closely related to our BMI. The larger your lean muscle mass, the more fat calories your muscles burn each day. This sends your metabolism higher. At the same time, your BMI should drop in proportion.

The higher your metabolism, the healthier you should be and the less likely you are to have a BMI over 25.

IB #6 describes how we have complete control over our personal metabolic rate and how we can raise it by eating a lean diet and exercising. You will also read how animal studies show that eating lean empowers your immunity.

Is Your Calorie-Burning Furnace Almost Extinguished?

The body's lean muscle mass is actually our calorie-burning furnace. But by age 30 most Americans have become so sedentary that the average person begins to lose 6 pounds of muscle with each decade. As our muscles become weak and flabby from lack of use, they atrophy and burn less fat. Our metabolism starts to drop and the body's fat stores begin to grow. As the years go by, the body's muscle mass becomes too small to burn off all the surplus calories we eat, and we develop a potbelly and begin to bulge out in all the wrong places.

The immune system thrives on a healthy body composition, that is, on a healthy ratio of lean muscle mass to body fat. The biological cause of most corpulence is loss of lean muscle mass due to lack of exercise, coupled with excessive deposits

163

of body fat through overeating calories and fat. Thus what we weigh is an inaccurate indicator of body health. The solution to being corpulent is not merely to lose pounds, but instead to focus on increasing muscle size and cutting fat out of the diet.

A Whole-Person Solution

In the final analysis obesity is a whole-person problem involving attitude as well as exercise and eating habits, and it requires a whole-person solution on the psychological, physical and nutritional levels to beat it. Trying to lose weight by merely cutting calories is almost always destined to fail.

Moreover, while aerobic exercise like brisk walking provides enough physical exertion to help restore some peoples' body composition to normal, for many others, brisk rhythmic exercise may not be enough.

Aerobic exercise certainly keeps our muscles in shape and it even causes a small increase in muscle size. But many people with stubborn fat require a combination of both aerobic *and* strength-building exercise before they can build back the original body muscles they had when they were younger. Their new muscles are then sufficiently large to gradually burn off their surplus weight—provided, of course, that they also eliminate the surplus fat and calories from their diet.

"Ideal Weight" Is an Obsolete Concept

Because of the new focus on body composition, the traditional tables of "ideal weight" developed by the Metropolitan Insurance Company and the USDA have become obsolete.

On January 1, 1996, the USDA released a revolutionary new version of these tables based on BMI. BMI replaces all previous weight tables because it provides an assessment of the health of your body in terms of the ratio between body muscle and body fat. It also provides a rough, but fairly accurate, guide to the probable vigor of your immuno-competence.

The BMI guidelines are published in a table in the revised *Dietary Guidelines for Americans*, which is available in most libraries and on the Internet. If you are still using an old ideal weight table, I recommend discarding it immediately. Today's ideal weights in terms of BMI are 10 to 15 percent below those of earlier years.

Despite the urgent need to shed surplus pounds, most Americans are becoming heavier, not lighter. Over the past decade, the average person has added an average of 8 pounds. One reason is that until 1996 Americans had been grossly misinformed about the level of their ideal weight. Since 1970, ideal weight levels had been repeatedly pushed upwards by flawed statistics based on insurance company mortality tables. Because smokers and people with cancer die younger, insurance tables showed that people lived longer when they weighed 10 to 15 pounds above their ideal weight. The old tables gave separate ideal weights for men and women and more permissive weights for people over 35.

New Guidelines for Normalizing Your Body's Composition

The new BMI guidelines ignore age and apply equally to both adult men and women. A table shows whether your weight is in the "healthy" range or whether you are "moder-

165

ately overweight" or "severely overweight." When your weight enters the "severely overweight" range, you have a growing risk of cancer and immuno-suppression (as well as heart disease and diabetes).

The new guidelines describe a weight range rather than pinpointing a specific ideal weight. For example, a weight between 140 to 187 pounds is described as healthy for a man or woman 6 feet tall. While this is adequate for general use, if you have a calculator handy, you can make a much more accurate assessment of the health of your body composition. All you need is your height in inches without shoes and your weight in pounds unclothed. With these two figures you can calculate your personal BMI in about two minutes. (Tip: It's best to weigh yourself as soon as you get up in the morning before you eat or drink anything.)

How to Calculate Your Personal Body Mass Index

Step 1. Multiply your weight in pounds by 705.
Step 2. Divide the result of step 1 by your height in inches.
Step 3. Then divide the result of step 2 by your height in inches.

For example, for a man or woman weighing 160 pounds and standing 5'5" in height (65 inches) the calculation is:

Step 1. 160 x 705 = 112,800
Step 2. 112,800/65 = 1735.4
Step 3. 1735.4/65 = 26.7

The resulting Body Mass Index is 26.7. To find out how healthy your body composition is, and to obtain a rough

166

guide to the vigor of your immune system, look your BMI up in the table below.

BMI Body Health and Immunity Assessment Guide

BMI Level	Body Health and Immunity Risk Assessment
20-22	Excellent body composition with ideal fat/muscle ratio. Optimal level of immuno-competence.
23-25	Good body composition with mildly elevated level of body fat. Vigorous level of immuno competence.
26-27	Moderately overweight. Fair body composition with fairly high level of body fat. Immuno-competence remains quite strong.
28 or over	Seriously overweight. Poor body composition with excessive body fat and too little muscle. Certain immune functions may be impaired.
32 or over	Severely overweight. Very poor body composition with a dangerously high level of body fat and a strong possibility of muscle atrophy. Function of immune system likely to be weak with declining ability to fight off infections and to recognize and destroy cancer cells.

If your BMI were 26.7, as in the example, you would probably appear moderately overweight and your immune system should still function well. But you would be perilously close to the borderline. Anyone with a BMI of 28 or over has an above-average risk of immune system impairment and should take immediate steps to adjust his or her BMI to under 25.

A No-Nonsense Weight-Loss Plan That Really Works

By now you have probably realized that this is an entirely new approach to weight loss. In fact, it's the *only* weight-loss plan that really works. You don't have to diet or count calories. But you do have to eat foods that are different from those you've probably been used to. And you will have to exert your muscles. If you're a woman who has been unable to lose weight, even by dieting plus aerobic exercise, the weight-loss plan that follows may require you to exert your muscles in a different way. *That's because the secret of normalizing your body composition lies in building up strong skeleletal muscles, not in trying to shed pounds by dieting.*

From here on, body composition is what counts, not body weight. Because muscle weighs more than fat and is more compact, you can restore a healthy body composition without actually losing much weight. However, even though you don't lose much weight, as you restore your BMI to a healthy level, you will have a superbly sculpted body. Your body will quickly begin to look better even if your weight remains the same.

How Abdominal Fat May Suppress Immunity

Millions of Americans try to eat their way out of stress or unhappiness by constantly snacking on sweet and fatty foods. As fat and calories pile up in the bloodstream, the adrenal glands release the stress hormones cortisol and adrenalin. Numerous studies have shown that cortisol is released in response to emotional stress. In conjunction with adrenalin, it then drives fat to the abdomen where it forms a potbelly. Meanwhile, any surplus calories are stored as fat over the rest of the body.

By way of proof, a study at Yale University of 41 overweight women aged 18 to 40 showed that those who carried their excess weight on the abdomen secreted significantly more cortisol when exposed to stress. Thus stress can determine where body fat is stored. In tests, cortisol has even been shown to relocate fat from the thighs to the abdomen.

It has also been well documented that cortisol directly suppresses the immune system. Thus a middle-age spread may well be an indicator of immuno-suppression.

Abdominal fat, also known as central or tummy fat, is particularly dangerous because it has been directly linked to several types of cancer, as well as to heart diseases, diabetes and other chronic diseases. One survey of women with breast cancer at the University of South Florida in Tampa found that they had 45 percent more deep abdominal fat than women without breast cancer.

How to Calculate Your Waist-to-Hip Ratio

A simple do-it-yourself test called the *waist-to-hip ratio* (WHR) reveals the extent of your belly fat and also possibly indicates a condition of immuno-suppression due to excessive stress. Here's how to do it.

Remove all clothing around your waist and hips.

1. Measure the smallest circumference around your waist at the slimmest point.
2. Measure the largest circumference around your buttocks at the widest part of your hips.

Just relax and breathe naturally while taking the measurements. Don't try to cheat by sucking in your abdomen or holding your breath.

Next, divide your waist size by your hip size.

For example, say you measure 36 inches at the slimmest part of your waist and 40 inches at the widest part of your hips. Dividing 36 by 40 equals 0.9. This is your waist-to-hip ratio and it indicates the extent of fat stored in your abdomen.

A ratio of 0.95 or lower is good for men.

A ratio of 0.8 or lower is good for women.

A higher WHR indicates an unhealthy level of body fat. If you have a higher ratio, it may indicate that stress is causing dietary fat to migrate to your middle. Central or abdominal fat above and around the waist may also indicate some degree of immuno-suppression. The higher the ratio, the greater is the possibility of impairment to your immuno-competence and the higher your risk of cancer or infections.

It's Time to Get Out of the La-Z-Boy

During studies in the early 1990s it was discovered that people with above-normal WHRs frequently have higher insulin levels. In lab tests, insulin appears to promote growth of breast cancer cells. The same series of studies also showed that postmenopausal women who accumulated fat above the waist (apple-shaped) were more prone to develop breast cancer than those who accumulated fat below the waist (pear shaped).

Abdominal or belly fat is rare in people of any age who exercise. To start with, exercise burns off surplus fat and calories. But people who exercise also have larger muscles and muscle is biologically active. Each pound of body muscle burns about 48 calories per day, even when resting, while body fat burns none. Any man or woman who has main-

tained his or her lean muscle mass through exercise is unlikely to have a BMI over 25.

People add weight when they put up their feet and stop
exercising. A few months of sedentary living will cause almost anyone's muscles to become flabby and weak. As our
muscles shrink, their mass becomes too small to burn off
the body's fat and calories. The result: Our metabolism
plummets while our BMI heads for the stratosphere.

Your BMI is a direct indicator of the ratio between your
muscle mass and body fat. But our present BMI is not something we're stuck with for life. We all have direct personal
control over our BMI. And provided we're willing to do what
it takes to succeed, every one of us can raise our metabolism
by rebalancing the muscle-to-fat composition of our bodies.

The secret to lowering your BMI to 25 or below—and
your waist-to-hip ratio to a healthy level—is outlined in the
8-step program below. Look up each of the Immune Boosters
listed below and follow the instructions for carrying them
out.

THE 8-STEP WEIGHT-LOSS AND IMMUNE BOOSTING PROGRAM

Step 1. Read, follow and practice IB #8: Unlock Your
Immune Power with Aerobic Exercise. Follow the instructions and begin to exercise aerobically for up to 45 minutes
or more three or more days each week.

Step 2. Read, adopt and practice IB #9: The Stronger
Your Muscles, the Stronger Your Immunity. Follow the instructions and begin to work out with strength-training machines or free weights three or more days each week for 45

171

minutes or longer. While there's nothing wrong with using abdominal exercises to flatten a bulging belly, aim to rebuild the lean muscle mass all over your body. Spot reducing seldom works. As you build up muscles in your arms, shoulders and legs, you are also helping to flatten your tummy.

Together, steps 1 and 2 should have you exercising six days a week as you alternate an aerobic workout one day with a strength-building workout the next.

Step 3. Read, adopt and practice IB #3: Cut Back on Foods That Cripple Your Immune System. Learn to identify foods that pile on fat and suppress your immunity, and cut them completely out of your diet.

Step 4. Read, adopt and practice IB #4: The One Diet That Does It All. Follow the instructions and begin eating foods that fight diseases up front so they don't have a chance to overload your immune system. These same foods also help maintain your body composition at its optimal level.

Step 5. Read, adopt and practice IB #6: Boost Your Immunity by Eating Lean. Learn how to eat smart and avoid the dozens of food traps that pile on the fat.

Step 6. Read, adopt and practice IBs #16 and #17 and visualize yourself as strong and lean. As we think, feel, say, and visualize, so we become.

Step 7. Read, adopt and practice IB #18: Defuse Depression with Cognitive Positivism, and learn how to keep stress and depression out of your life.

Step 8. Every 14 days recalculate your BMI and WHR (and also your metabolism) and record your progress in a diary. Even a small success can boost your enabling effect and motivation. Also keep track of how you look and feel. In 2 or 3 weeks, many people with poor body composition begin to look and feel better than they have in years. As these benefits appear, your healing-regeneration system kicks in, and your immuno-competence begins to soar.

Revitalizing Your Body Is Simpler Than It Sounds

If all that sounds overwhelming, consider this. Three of the Immune Boosters are about nutrition so you only have to learn the principles of sound nutrition once. Nor do you have to commence everything immediately. In the beginning, focus on starting the exercise routines and begin to cut the fat out of your diet. Start in at a level that won't tax you and increase gradually thereafter.

However, if you're female and have a problem with stubborn fat, you may have to exercise more than you expected. Twenty minutes of walking three times a week isn't enough to burn off body fat. It's much easier for men to lose weight through exercise because they have larger muscles to begin with. And muscle is what drives up metabolism and consumes fat.

Therefore, to get your BMI below 25, you must be willing to use your mind and muscles to do what it takes to succeed. That means working out on strength-building equipment, exercising aerobically at a pace brisk enough to make you perspire and following the guidelines for getting the fat out of your diet.

It should all become much easier if you also practice IB #17 and learn to "see" yourself as slender and lean. Adopting the stress management techniques in IB #18 also helps.

Conquer Obesity Without Drugs or Dieting

If that sounds like too many things to have to do, the alternatives are either appetite-suppressing drugs or dieting. For six people out of ten, diet pills do work, at least to some extent. They inhibit food cravings by releasing serotonin, a soothing neurotransmitter into the brain. The catch is that

173

the drugs work only when used in conjunction with a low-fat diet and exercise. Once you adopt a low-fat diet and exercise routine like that in the 8-step program just described, who needs drugs anyway?

In September 1997, the FDA acted to withdraw two of the most popular diet drugs. The reason: Tests showed that the drugs caused heart valve damage in 30 percent of users. Other diet drugs that manipulate brain chemistry may also cause long-term side effects like reduced libido, depression or memory impairment. That's in addition to such short-term side effects as drowsiness, dry mouth or diarrhea. Of course, the moment you stop taking these drugs, your weight shoots back up. When you add it all up, losing weight by taking diet drugs doesn't sound too exciting.

Anyone who has read this book so far knows that dieting is futile. Yet millions of women, and some men, continue to persist in trying to lose weight through calorie restriction alone. Few realize that, as a low-calorie diet reduces metabolism, the body reads this as a threat of approaching starvation. Instead of losing fat, the body catabolizes its own muscle tissue for fuel, while conserving its fat stores and hoarding even more.

The result is a lower percentage of lean muscle mass and a higher percentage of body fat. Incredibly, most diets actually raise the BMI instead of lowering it. Rather than losing fat, the body adds more fat while muscle tissue fades away. When we diet through calorie restriction (by cutting carbohydrates), one-third of all weight loss is due to loss of lean muscle mass, while most of the remainder is due to loss of body fluid.

By contrast, when we exercise aerobically or with strength-building equipment, 100 percent of the weight we lose is pure body fat. Lean muscle mass is our body's calorie-burning furnace and the only way to turn it on is by exercise. Once we adopt the 8-step program just described, our body's muscle mass will gradually burn away our reserves of stored fat while our BMI drops to 25 or below.

IMMUNE BOOSTER #6: **Boost Your Immunity by Eating Lean**

Results from scores of studies across the globe all strongly suggest that what we eat and how much play an important role in bolstering immunity.

For example, most people who eat the Standard American Diet consume so much fat and protein, and so few fruits and vegetables, that one-third of the American population is overweight and another one-third is obese. Scores of studies have demonstrated that being overweight suppresses immunity and promotes the development of diseases such as cancer that then overburden the immune system and weaken it still more.

For example, in 1996 the American Cancer Society's guidelines identified obesity as contributing to increased risk of cancer of the colon, endometrium, kidney, prostate and rectum, and breast cancer among postmenopausal women. Excess body fat increases production of estrogen in women and of testosterone in men, thus heightening the risk of both breast and prostate cancer.

Dozens of experiments on rats and mice have clearly shown that when fed a lean diet—low in fat and calories—they were markedly more resistant to cancer and infections. Tests on other lab animals indicated that eating fewer calories and less fat keeps the thymus gland active longer and reduces activity of T-suppressor cells. The result: The im-

175

mune system responds more vigorously to infections and cancer cells.

Cutting Back on Fat May Downsize a Tumor

Other experiments have shown that eating fewer fat calories may slow or even stop growth of a small tumor already in place. For instance, a study by Dr. William Fair, a surgeon at Memorial Sloan-Kettering Cancer Center, New York, found that when fat in the diet of mice injected with human prostate cancer cells was cut back to 20 percent or less of their calories, the tumors stopped growing.

The tumors were still there, but growth had ceased. If growth of prostate cancer can be slowed or stopped, it almost amounts to a cure. And in locations like the prostate gland, indications are that tumor growth may indeed be slowed or stopped by how and what we eat.

Further confirmation comes from the work of Dr. Robert Good, a prominent immunologist and former director of Memorial Sloan-Kettering Cancer Center. Back in the 1980s, Dr. Good showed that a diet high in calories can speed up shrinkage of the thymus gland, the vital organ that processes new T-cells. A deficiency of T-cells may seriously suppress the immune system and distort its balance. And the more a person is overweight, the more likely this is to happen.

These findings recently prompted CapCure, the world's largest private funding source for prostate cancer research, to launch a major nutritional project to determine if diet therapy really can help men with advanced prostate cancer. Although final proof may take several years, preliminary indications support the concept that prostate cancer tumor

176

growth is fueled by the high-fat Western diet and that it can be prevented, slowed or stopped by switching to a low-fat, plant-based diet similar to that described in IB #4. By adopting IB #4: The One Diet That Does It All, any man with prostate cancer given the option of "watchful waiting" by his physician, might well avoid ever having to undergo further treatment.

Overeating Suppresses Immunity

Ongoing studies by Roy C. Walford, Ph.D., an immunologist at UCLA, have confirmed that people who eat a lean diet and avoid overeating have immune systems that are consistently stronger than those of the general public.

Using lab animals, Dr. Walford found that overeating causes atrophy of the thymus gland, leading to premature weakening of the immune system. When calorie intake was reduced by one-third, while intake of all essential vitamins and minerals was maintained, the decline in immuno-competence due to aging was so retarded that many animals far outlived their normal life expectancies.

A similar study by Dr. Richard Weindruch of the National Institutes on Aging found that animals fed 50 percent fewer calories also had stronger immune systems and a lower incidence of diseases compared with those fed normal numbers of calories. Weindruch believes that calorie restriction may preserve certain immune system components, particularly the thymus gland which regulates production of T-cells.

Observations of men who were light eaters have also shown that the immune system may remain actively resistant to cancer and infections until well past the century mark. Further support comes from a study of nine anorexic volun-

177

teers, each of whom showed a normal-to-strong response on some immune tests, while six had not had a single infection during the previous year.

Obviously, it isn't necessary to become anorexic to improve immunity. In fact, Weindruch has cautioned against any form of self-starvation or calorie deprivation because nutritional deficiencies could become a problem. It's important to note that in all the studies showing improved immunity due to a lean diet, none of the lab animals was malnourished. All received a full daily quota of vitamins, minerals and other essential nutrients. Only calorie intake was cut.

Moreover, both Drs. Walford and Weindruch have become so convinced by the results of their studies that both follow diets that build increased immune protection through a healthy level of body leanness.

Many researchers today believe that we can significantly upgrade our immune systems without undergoing the draconion calorie cuts used in lab animal studies. Instead, they suggest that we simply adopt the following three steps for healthier eating:

1. Eat only as many calories as our metabolism needs.
2. Eat a diet low in fat and high in fiber.
3. Cut back on animal protein and replace it with protein from plant foods.

Eat Only As Many Calories As Your Metabolism Needs

So how many calories does your metabolism need? Until recently, calculating your metabolism was difficult and expensive. But a new simple formula developed by Dr. C.

178

Wayne Calloway, an obesity specialist at George Washington University, Washington, D.C., allows anyone with a pocket calculator to calculate his or her personal metabolism in just a few minutes.

First, here's how to calculate your resting metabolism, that is, the number of calories your body-mind uses each 24 hours while completely at rest.

MEN

Step 1. Multiply your height in inches by 12.7.
Step 2. Multiply your weight in pounds by 6.3.
Step 3. Add these two numbers and then add 66.
Step 4. Multiply your age by 6.8.
Step 5. Subtract the result of step 4 from step 3.
The result is your resting rate of metabolism.

WOMEN

Step 1. Multiply your height in inches by 4.7.
Step 2. Multiply your weight in pounds by 4.3.
Step 3. Add these numbers and then add 655.
Step 4. Multiply your age by 4.7.
Step 5. Subtract the result of step 4 from step 3.
The result is your resting rate of metabolism.

Now to calculate your nonresting metabolism, all you need do is multiply your resting metabolic rate by one of the factors below. Pick the one that best fits your activity level.

1. If you are totally at rest all day, multiply by 1.2.
2. If you are only mildly active, multiply by 1.3.

179

3. If you exercise three to four times a week, multiply by 1.4.
4. If you exercise actively four or more times a week, multiply by 1.6.
5. If you are very active and exercise vigorously for one hour or more almost daily, multiply by 1.8.

Here's an example. George is 56 years old and is 72 inches tall, he weighs 180 pounds, and he exercises actively four or more times a week.

Step 1. 72 x 12.7 = 914.4
Step 2. 180 x 6.3 = 1134
Step 3. 914.4 + 1134 + 66 = 2114.4
Step 4. 56 x 6.8 = 380.8
Step 5. 2114.4–380.8 = 1733.6

George's resting metabolic rate is 1733.6 calories per 24 hours. Since his activity level is 4, he multiplies 1733.6 by 1.6. Thus his nonresting metabolic rate is 2773.76 calories per 24 hours.

Regulate Your Body's Fat Furnace

By calculating your nonresting metabolic rate once each month, you can easily keep track of any increase. While you may think that changing something like your body's metabolism is completely beyond your control, that's not true. Changing our metabolism for the better is something we can all accomplish if we're willing to do what it takes to succeed.

The higher your metabolism, the more body fat it burns and the less likely you are to be overweight. IB #5 describes how to raise your metabolism through physical activity. As the remainder of this Immune Booster shows, you can also increase it by improving your diet and eating habits.

But most of all, right now, your nonresting metabolic rate tells exactly how many calories you can eat at your present level of activity without gaining weight. Eat fewer calories than your metabolic rate and your weight should start to drop. Eat more, and your weight is likely to start creeping up.

Yet trying to count the number of calories of food you consume each day is a cumbersome and time-consuming task. A far simpler way is to double the amount of foods you eat that grow on plants and halve the amount of meat, poultry, dairy products (except plain nonfat), eggs, fats and oils. Aim to eat at least six servings daily of raw or cooked vegetables, three or more servings of fruit, 6 to 11 servings of whole grains and one or more servings of legumes. This provides a total of 16 or more servings of unprocessed plant foods each day. After that, the more plant-based foods and the fewer flesh foods, dairy products (except plain nonfat), eggs, oils and fats you eat, the sooner your BMI will reach a healthy level.

If your BMI is above 25, this one step should bring your total calorie intake from food far closer to your nonresting metabolic rate than it probably is right now. By taking that step, you should be very close to eating a completely plant-based diet. That means you'll be eating approximately the same "lean diet" that has given the immune system a dramatic boost in literally hundreds of animal and human studies.

Fewer Pounds Boosts Immunity

For example, in 1993 when the blood of 19 Japanese men and women was analyzed for immune reactions, it was found that being overweight dangerously weakened the response of T-cells. After participants had each lowered their weight by an average of 50 pounds, the defensive powers of their T-cells almost doubled.

Other studies have shown that anyone who has gained 10 to 15 pounds since age 21, or whose waistline has increased by 2 to 3 inches, has a much higher risk of cancer and of immuno-suppression. Men with cancer of the prostate or testes and women with cancer of the breast or ovaries have appeared to benefit from a reduced intake of calories, animal protein and fat. Partly, that's because hormonal cancers such as these are most common in overweight people.

Considerable evidence exists to suggest that cutting back on calories until your BMI is 25 or lower may impede development of new tumors and retard growth of existing ones, especially in the prostate. If your BMI drops below 25, that's even better. But never allow your BMI to go below the 20 to 21 range. A BMI of 19 or lower could compromise your immunity (see IB #5).

A New Way to Look at Food

Switching to a plant-based diet is a whole lot easier when we learn to rethink what a plate of food looks like. Meat or chicken doesn't have to be the centerpiece of every dish. We can get the same taste enjoyment from plant foods as from meat, chicken or eggs. And fruit is often tastier than ice cream.

Most problems we have with cutting back on calories, fat or protein have more to do with the foods we eat with than with taste. Would you offer your friends and family a meatless dish at a dinner party, even though the vegetables and grains were based on a delicious recipe from India or Japan? Probably not, and the reason is that these foods aren't socially acceptable in our affluent society. Most Americans regard a plant-based diet as frugal and restrictive. In fact, millions of Americans still regard beans and rice as peasant food, fit only for people in Third World countries.

Yet if you're really serious about upgrading your immunity, eating foods that grow on plants is the ideal way to achieve the "lean diet" that studies show can help supercharge your immune system.

You don't have to switch to a plant-based diet in a single day. Doing so could fill your digestive tract with so much unfamiliar fiber that you could experience discomfort. So add one new fruit, vegetable or grain every few days while you drop a comparable amount of meat, poultry and other inappropriate foods.

Eating Out: A Giant Fat Trap

The important thing is to stay in control of what you eat and don't let food control you. Be particularly watchful when eating with friends or family or at a restaurant. Surveys show that fewer than half of all Americans keep nutrition in mind when eating out. Once faced with a choice of foods, most people forget about their good intentions. Given a choice between a baked potato and French fries, 80 percent of people in one survey chose the fries.

Obviously, you can make wise food choices more easily in a restaurant that has a buffet-type salad bar. Simply order "soup and salad" and stick to low-fat dressings. Otherwise, never go to a restaurant hungry. Surveys show that during the first 10 minutes after being seated in a restaurant, a hungry person devours almost anything the waiter brings, whether it's bread and rolls, hors d'oeuvres or anything else.

You can distance yourself from this type of overeating by eating a small salad or a piece of fruit with yogurt *before* you leave home.

Watch out for oversized servings in restaurants. Observers report that American restaurants serve meals that are 25 percent larger than a decade ago. Muffins and bagels are twice the size they were 10 years ago, and many sandwiches are loaded with 5 to 8 ounces of meat. Others are filled with processed meats and thick slabs of hard cheese.

The Sandwich Trap

Sandwiches can be one of the worst fat traps. It's hard to tell what any sandwich may contain. Vegetarian sandwiches can be made with whole wheat bread or pita and appear to be stuffed with sprouts, but they can still contain a thick slab of fat-laden cheese. A tuna sandwich with mayo often contains more fat than a Big Mac. It's safest to fill your own sandwiches from a salad bar, using either whole wheat bread or pita.

Some surveys show that when we eat with friends or relatives whom we know well, we tend to eat 50 percent more food than when we eat with strangers or alone. And when we eat a low-fat version of any food, we tend, on average, to eat 25 percent more of it.

From TV commercials to parties, social events and restaurant eating, we are constantly being exhorted to overeat. Giving in to any such food traps could start your immunity heading south.

Why America's Weight Is Out of Control

One giant food trap is even more destructive to our immunity. That's eating when we're not really hungry. Millions of Americans, particularly women, use food as a tranquilizer whenever they feel bored, worried, unhappy or pressured or when they're feeling anxious, lonely or unloved. Whenever we eat a candy bar, ice cream or chocolate or drink a sugar-filled soda, it triggers an immediate rise in our blood sugar level that brings temporary relief from our sagging emotions.

Surveys show that whenever we eat for purely psychological reasons—to relieve stress or negative feelings—we are responding to cues such as the aroma, texture, crunchiness or sizzle of food. These cues trigger childhood memories of when Mom gave us sweet or fatty foods to make us feel content and happy.

As adults, we crave those same pleasant feelings and memories so we crave the same sweet or fatty foods that pacified us as kids. And millions of us overeat these foods to the point of substance abuse. We become as addicted to these foods as an alcoholic is to liquor or a smoker is to cigarettes.

While these foods relieve stress by piling up fat and calories in the bloodstream, the adrenal glands are releasing the stress hormones cortisol (a powerful immuno-suppressant) and adrenaline. Working together, these hormones cause the fat just eaten to migrate to the waistline where it forms a pot belly. Meanwhile, other surplus calories are stored as fat all over the body.

Once we develop an addiction to high-fat, high-calorie binge foods, certain events may trigger a craving. While watching TV or a ball game, we may binge on cheese snacks or potato chips, totally unaware of how much we are eating.

How to Beat a Craving for Binge Foods

As soon as a craving arises, take ten slow, deep breaths. Realize that you aren't actually hungry. You don't really need the potato chips, cheese snack or ice cream. You simply crave the crunchiness or the creamy texture and the memories they bring back.

Then right away do something that is incompatible with eating. Run in place for five minutes or take a quick walk around the block. Within a few minutes, the craving should subside. The realization that much of our eating is purely psychological, and not because we're hungry, is usually sufficient to enable most of us to break this form of substance abuse.

Six Ways to Prevent Future Binging

1. Make a list of your favorite binge foods such as ice cream, cookies, cakes, doughnuts, potato chips, crackers, cheese, cheese snacks, candies, chocolate, pizza or fried chicken. Women tend to prefer sweet fats, while men prefer salty fats like French fries, hot dogs or pepperoni.

2. Recognize that you binge on these problem foods in response to a trigger event or situation. So make a list of all the situations that cause you to head for the refrigerator. Typical trigger situations are watching TV, writing creatively, working on a report, socializing at a party, eating in a restaurant or talking on the phone. And, of course, feeling pressured, bored, worried, unhappy, anxious, lonely or unloved.

3. Stop buying these binge foods so they're out of reach. Replace them with healthier, low-fat snacks like plain air-popped popcorn, celery, carrot sticks, rice cakes or fruit. If

186

you do buy a binge food, purchase only the smallest amount so that you cannot keep on eating.

4. Avoid eating during or immediately after a trigger situation. For instance, never eat while standing or when on the phone. Except for fruits, vegetables or other healthy low-fat snacks, avoid finger foods at social gatherings. If you do pick them up, only use your nondominant hand. Never send out for food if you can avoid it. And never again let a binge food control you to the point where you can't control the amount you eat.

5. Tests on people who are compulsive overeaters show that you can get as much pleasure from eating a very small amount of a binge food as from gobbling down a large amount. First, set aside a small portion, or just a single piece, of the food you will eat and understand that this is *all* you will eat. Then take a small piece of the food, close your eyes and smell it. Bite into it slowly and enjoy a maximum taste sensation as you chew it and it gradually dissolves. Experience the texture of the food and the nuances of its flavors. Focus your entire attention on what you are eating and extract every moment of pleasure from it. It should take about 5 minutes to eat a small piece in this way. Many people report that this focused taste experience provides more actual eating pleasure than gobbling down a whole bag of chips or pint of ice cream.

6. Staying focused on food while eating it is also known as mindfulness. Practicing mindfulness while eating forces you to be aware of, and to think about, your food. Eating while you read, talk to someone or watch TV can distract you from your food and cause you to binge or overeat. Each of these distractions dilutes your experience of taste and causes you to lose track of the amount you have eaten.

By staying focused on your food, you will notice, as the

187

meal progresses, that the intensity of taste diminishes because our olfactory receptors are saturated. In that case, why keep on eating?

To avoid overeating and binging, chew your food for twice the normal time. And eat with your eyes closed to maximize the taste experience. Another tip: Don't eat leftovers cold. Warming them will double their taste.

Grazing: The New Way to Lose Weight Without Dieting

Several small studies have shown that when overweight people switch to a "grazing" routine, they often lose an average of 2 pounds per week without cutting calories. Grazing means dividing your regular three meals into either six or nine mini-meals and eating them at more frequent intervals throughout the day. You continue to eat the same quantity of food, and the same number of calories, as you normally would in three main meals. But by breaking each main meal into two or three mini-meals, you reduce the fat storage that occurs when you eat three full-sized meals each day.

This has a very simple explanation: Our early ancestors seldom ate a full meal. Instead, they grazed, snacking on fruits, nuts, berries and tubers they gathered. Since our digestive systems have hardly changed in tens of thousands of years, grazing still works well today. For it to work, though, we must graze on plant foods, just as our ancestors did, eating high-fiber, low-fat vegetables, fruits, whole grains, legumes, nuts and seeds.

The easiest way for the average working person to begin grazing is to eat hot mini-meals at home and take snacks for midmorning and midafternoon breaks and at lunchtime.

Typical mini-meals could consist of plain air-popped popcorn, rice cakes, a banana or cucumber sandwich, sunflower seeds and raisins, an apple or other fruit or celery and carrot sticks.

Once a day, or once a week, reward yourself with a fruit cocktail, consisting of a mango, persimmon, banana, pear, grapes or kiwi fruit topped with a dab of plain nonfat yogurt.

Can Fasting Help Immunity?

If cutting back on calories gives the immune system a lift, wouldn't a fast work even better?

Considerable evidence shows that a full or partial fast does send our immunity soaring. During famines in Africa, people who were half-starved had less TB and malaria than their better-fed counterparts in refugee camps. When a group of overweight people fasted at the University of Pittsburgh School of Medicine, researchers found a marked increase in lymphocyte count. Several animal studies have also shown that rodents increased resistance to infections when deprived of food for two or three days.

But the benefit is short-lived so fasting is *not* the way to boost immunity. After several days without food, complications occur in the body that stress the kidneys and decrease blood volume. People with diabetes, low blood sugar or stomach ulcers should never fast.

If you're healthy, it's OK to fast for 24 hours, provided you drink plenty of water. But in some people a longer fast can lead to confusion or poor memory and, in diabetics, to possible coma and death.

189

Why High-Protein, Low-Carbohydrate Diets Don't Work

All foods basically consist of carbohydrates, fat and protein. Nutritionists often describe the components of a diet with a three-figure code: 64/16/20, meaning that, in terms of calories, 64 percent of a person's diet consists of carbohydrates, 16 percent is fat and 20 percent is protein. A 64/16/20 diet is high in carbohydrates, low in fat and provides just about the right amount of protein.

Nowadays, however, radical new weight-loss programs advocate cutting carbohydrate intake while increasing the intake of fat and protein. These programs typically suggest a 40/25/35 configuration, and people who eat this way often manage to lose a few pounds.

But the flaw in this diet is the misuse of the word "carbohydrates." To most people, "carbohydrate" means bread, sugar, sweeteners, pasta, perhaps potatoes, and all the cakes, pastries, cookies and other foods made from refined or simple carbohydrates. The high-protein weight-loss school refers to this type of carbohydrate as "concentrated carbohydrate." This description is apt because refined carbohydrates consist of nothing but a concentration of empty calories.

Eat the Right Carbohydrates

Most people don't realize it, but there are "good" and "bad" carbohydrates. For starters, every food that grows on a plant is basically a carbohydrate. From lettuce to apples, broccoli, citrus fruits, carrots, grapes, legumes, melons, whole grains, seeds and nuts, every food that grows on a plant consists primarily of carbohydrate.

190

Some, like avocadoes, beans, grains, nuts and seeds also contain some fat, primarily the harmless monounsaturated variety. These foods also contain some protein.

But no single plant food provides the kind of whole, complete protein that exists in foods of animal origin. However, when beans and grains are eaten together, the combination provides a whole protein comparable in quality with that obtained from animal foods.

Avoid "Bad" Carbohydrates

"Bad" carbohydrates are also known as simple, refined or concentrated carbohydrates. They are produced when a plant food such as grain, rice or sugar is milled, stripped of its germ and cellulose walls and transformed into white flour, rice or sugar. The sole reason for refining carbohydrates is to increase shelf life, thus allowing the food industry to realize greater profits.

Never forget that all types of sweeteners are also refined carbohydrates, including honey, molasses, brown sugar, extracted fructose and beet sugar, dextrose, malt, galactose, sorghum, sorbitol, xylose and, lastly, *all forms of alcohol*. Dried fruits, though high in fiber, contain a high concentration of sucrose and should be eaten in limited quantities.

Since they lack cell walls, refined carbohydrates are rapidly absorbed by the digestive system, sending a flood of sugar into the bloodstream that sets blood sugar and insulin levels soaring.

Though the body's need for refined carbohydrates is zero, manufacturers include these nutrient-deprived carbohydrates in virtually every type of prepared, processed, manufactured and canned food. "Bad" carbohydrates abound in commer-

191

cial cakes, pies, pastries, doughnuts and just about all baked goods.

Avoid Those Empty, Denuded Carbohydrates

One reason why so many of us are deficient in fiber is that the grains we do eat consist largely of white or refined wheat flour. In most supermarket breads and baked goods, white flour is the principal ingredient. Though the label on a loaf of white bread may list the first ingredient as "wheat flour," "unbleached wheat flour" or "unbleached enriched wheat flour," all are pseudonyms for refined white flour from which most of the germ and fiber have been stripped away.

Refining destroys 80 percent of all the fiber in wheat and leaches out most of the nutrients, including almost all the chromium, copper, folic acid, magnesium, manganese, zinc, vitamins B6 and E and just about all the phytomins, antioxidants and anticarcinogens.

Most white bread has the consistency of cotton and tastes like cardboard. To beef up the taste, refined sugar or corn syrup is often added as the second or third ingredient. Then, after thoroughly denuding the bread, some manufacturers try to add back three of the B vitamins and iron. Others attempt to restore the lost fiber by adding back heavily processed cellulose which is nutritionally worthless.

To avoid the refined carbohydrate trap, I recommend buying only bread that is labeled "100 percent whole wheat" or that is made entirely of oats, other whole grain flours or sprouted wheat. Bread labeled merely "whole wheat" may list whole wheat as the first ingredient, but it can also contain sizable amounts of refined carbohydrates as well. Most breads sold in health food stores have a full quota of fiber

192

and other nutrients. But you must read the labels carefully on supermarket breads. For instance, most commercial pumpernickel bread is made by adding caramel coloring to a mix of white and rye flour.

Naturally, all the drawbacks of white bread and sugar are equally applicable to white flour. Never use it for baking if whole wheat flour is available. Nor should you use white rice if brown rice can be had.

Eat Only Top-Notch Carbohydrates

"Good" carbohydrates, also known as complex carbohydrates, refer to any plant food still in the same whole, unprocessed, unfragmented and unrefined state in which it grew in nature. In this natural, unchanged condition, the still-living cells are enclosed in a membrane of cellulose. Most complex carbohydrates such as beans, grains, fruits, seeds or nuts will grow if planted in the ground. Also classified as complex carbohydrates are mildly processed grains like whole wheat flour and coarse-cut oatmeal, which retain many qualities of live foods during their short shelf life.

Complex carbohydrates are not exceptionally high in calories. A medium-sized potato has only 100 calories, but 300 if we fry it or plaster it with butter or sour cream. Yet millions of people still believe erroneously that plain baked potatoes or corn tortillas are fattening. Indeed, they are not. Often enough, it's what we put on complex carbohydrates that makes plant foods seem high in calories.

Though it may take several hours to digest and release their calories, complex carbohydrates are still the ideal high-energy food. When fresh fruits or vegetables are not available, plain frozen or canned ones may be used instead.

193

Complex carbohydrates are the only foods to contain any appreciable amount of fiber. Among complex carbohydrates with the highest fiber content are apples, barley, beans, carrots, citrus fruits, potatoes, prunes and sweet potatoes. "Good" carbohydrates like these fill you up without overloading the body with surplus calories, and they also dampen the insulin response.

The Flawed Theory of Insulin Resistance

If you examine them closely, you'll find that the high-protein weight-loss plans are slanted at people who eat only "bad" carbohydrates and who never exercise. Quite correctly, the authors of these plans claim that concentrated carbohydrates stimulate insulin secretion that causes the body to store fat. The more refined a carbohydrate is, the faster it is swept into the bloodstream and the more it elevates the body's insulin level. Elevated insulin levels then cause the body to store fat.

This is also the principle behind insulin resistance, another weight-loss concept based on cutting back on carbohydrates. The insulin resistance theory swept the country in the mid-1990s, causing millions of people to believe they had a genetic fat-burning impairment that they could do nothing about. Insulin resistance weight-loss plans merely cut back on carbohydrates and added fat. But the high-protein weight-loss plans went a step further and increased protein as well. Both are based on the following scenario.

During periods of abundance, the bodies of our early ancestors stored surplus calories in layers of fat as insurance against future food shortages. While early humans certainly did scavenge and hunt wild game, the meat's fat content was low and the bulk of people's diet consisted of foods that grow on plants—in other words, complex carbohydrates. (Refined carbohydrates such as white flour and sugar were unknown until just over a century ago.)

To transform a complex carbohydrate into energy and to store it in the muscles and the body's fat layers, the pancreas must secrete the hormone insulin.

How to Make Insulin Resistance Disappear

According to the insulin resistance theory, during periods of food abundance—which never ends in modern America—the pancreas overproduces insulin to convert carbohydrates into muscle energy and fat. Much of the carbohydrates we eat— especially refined carbohydrates—then end up adding to our fat reserves. Since modern humans are rarely, if ever, faced with a food shortage, these fat stores are never used. They remain permanently as unsightly flab on the abdomen, buttocks and thighs.

When we cut back on fat and eat more carbohydrates in an effort to lose weight, so much extra insulin is needed that the pancreas is swiftly overloaded, often to the point of burnout. Reaching this condition translates into a greatly increased risk of diabetes or heart disease.

For millions of Americans in the mid-1990s, the insulin resistance theory merely confirmed what they'd believed all along: that being overweight was beyond their control. After all, how can you lower the fat content of your diet if doing so places you at risk for a life-threatening disease?

While these facts are biologically sound, many weight-loss experts consider this theory extremely controversial—and a superb excuse for millions of people to continue eating a high-fat diet.

For starters, the insulin resistance theory totally ignores

195

any need for exercise. Virtually all bona fide cases of insulin resistance exist in people with flabby, atrophied muscles who haven't exercised in at least a decade. When people who are really insulin resistant rebuild their muscles with exercise, their new, larger muscles can store far more energy from carbohydrate foods. Larger muscles then give a powerful boost to their metabolism by burning far more calories every hour of every day.

When hundreds of additional calories are burned by aerobic exercise, the body's need for insulin is drastically reduced. Insulin resistance then disappears.

In any case, eating a high proportion of foods from carbohydrates does *not* make a person who is insulin resistant overweight. To become overweight, you must consume more calories than your nonresting metabolic rate.

Cutting Back on Carbohydrates Is Poor Advice

Furthermore, it's important to note that digesting complex carbohydrates consumes 25 calories per 100 calories of plant-based foods versus only 3 calories to digest 100 calories of fat. Therefore the more fat you eat, the lower your metabolism drops. And the more plant-based foods you eat, the more calories you burn to digest them and the higher your metabolism soars.

As you read in IB #5, the solution to insulin resistance is not to cut back on plant-based foods while eating more fat and protein. The answer is to lower your Body Mass Index by building up your muscles with a combination of aerobic and strength-building exercises while, at the same time, cutting back on dietary fat and eating more complex carbohydrates.

After analyzing various high-protein weight-loss plans, researchers from several leading university medical centers separately concluded that any weight loss that may occur is due entirely to the restriction of calories (caused by the low carbohydrate intake) and to water loss (explained below). The high-protein part of the diet simply prevents hunger pangs.

When eaten, each gram of carbohydrate binds with 3 grams of water in the body. So when we cut back on dietary carbohydrate, we lose three times as much weight in water. Further, since carbohydrate energy is stored in muscles, cutting back on carbohydrates leaves you with a lower muscle weight and proportionately more fat.

You Don't Lose Fat on a Low-Carbohydrate Diet

Whatever weight is actually lost through these plans consists primarily of water and muscle, not fat. Researchers also discovered that a low carbohydrate diet can adversely affect the emotions and increase the likelihood of bone loss.

The plans simply do not provide sufficient energy for exercise. And by cutting back on carbohydrates, they rob you of all the fiber, vitamins, minerals, phytomins, antioxidants and anticarcinogens available only in complex carbohydrates.

Meanwhile, the high-fat content promotes an avalanche of destructive free radicals. Several prominent nutritionists have described these high-protein diets as a step back into the Dark Ages of the 1950s when diets high in fat and protein launched an epidemic of cancer and heart disease.

It must be abundantly clear by now that carbohydrate-cutting weight-loss plans are only for people who eat substantial amounts of refined carbohydrates and who never exer-

197

cise. You can easily beat the insulin resistance trap by refusing to eat refined carbohydrates. While these "bad" refined carbohydrates send your insulin levels skywards, the "good" complex carbohydrates lead to a drop in insulin levels.

Real complex carbohydrate foods like fruits, vegetables, whole grains, legumes, nuts and seeds fill you up quickly without filling you with calories. The average plant-based meal will have you feeling full well before you have consumed 500 calories.

Nonfat Doesn't Mean Nonfattening

Millions of people have cut out red meat, fried and other fat-laden foods and replaced them with nonfat, fat-free or low-fat versions in the belief that they'll stop gaining weight.

Manufacturers may have taken the fat out of nonfat foods, but in most cases, they've simply replaced the fat calories with the same number of calories from refined carbohydrates, primarily sugar. Today, many fat-free foods contain just as many calories as before the fat was removed.

Certainly, calories from dietary fat turn into body fat faster than calories from carbohydrates. And dietary fat is more likely to migrate to belly, buttocks and thighs. But surplus calories from carbohydrates—especially refined carbohydrates—can also end up as body fat if we eat enough of them.

You can bypass this common food trap by replacing high-fat foods, not with low-fat versions, but with more fruits, vegetables, whole grains, legumes and a few nuts and seeds. Even then, to help lose body fat, it's best to go easy on such fat-containing plant foods as avocadoes, beans, nuts and seeds, at least until your BMI has dropped to 25 or below. I also suggest going easy on olive, canola and flaxseed oils. While these monounsaturated oils rarely promote free radicals, cancer or heart disease, they are still 100 percent pure fat.

Are There Any Good Fats?

The answer is yes and they're known as essential fatty acids, or EFAs, because our bodies cannot make them. EFAs play a vital role in regulating the immune response, and they are precursors of key hormones called *prostanoids* which cells use in communicating with each other.

There are only two EFAs:

Linoleic acid, an omega-6 fatty acid
Alpha-Linolenic acid, an omega-3 fatty acid

For our EFAs to be complete, we need both the omega-3 and omega-6 fatty acids. For this reason, many people believe that flaxseed oil is the one best source of both EFAs. One to two tablespoons daily mixed with food should ensure an ample supply of essential fatty acids.

These essential fats abound in soybeans and soybean products, in sunflower and sesame seeds, in nuts—especially almonds, filberts and walnuts—in green leafy vegetables and in canola, olive and flaxseed oils. To ensure that the EFAs are not destroyed during extraction, vegetable oils should be expeller-pressed and nonprocessed.

How Do Other Fats Affect the Immune System?

Among the four other types of fat, polyunsaturated vegetable oils (such as corn, safflower, soybean or sunflower oil) appear to enhance production of certain prostaglandins which may suppress the immune system.

Some years ago Dr. Michael Bennet and colleagues at the University of Texas Southwest Medical Center found that mice fed polyunsaturated safflower oil made a poor showing on most immune tests, while others fed saturated fats did little better. In contrast, mice fed 30 percent of their calories from a monounsaturated fat (olive oil) had good responses to most, though not quite all, immune tests.

However, the big surprise was that animals fed a low-fat diet, in which no more than 16 percent of calories were supplied by fat, showed a consistent and perfectly normal immune system, regardless of which type of fat they were fed.

When the results of these and similar studies are put together, it seems safe to assume that when animals are fed a diet rich in polyunsaturated fat, their immune systems become weaker than animals who are fed only negligable amounts of these fats. In fact, many lab animal studies show that a large amount of polyunsaturated fat in the diet has led to an increase in tumorigenesis.

Since Americans, on average, derive only about 8 percent of their calories from polyunsaturated fats (and up to 25 percent from saturated fats), the results of these animal studies may not be directly extrapolated to humans. Nonetheless, *they cannot be ignored.* For example, the Japanese who until recently ate a low-fat diet and obtained most of their fats from grains and legumes had one of the lowest cancer rates on earth.

For anyone seeking peak immunity, these animal studies

200

provide strong support for using olive or canola oils for cooking. They also strongly suggest keeping calories from all fats below 16 percent of total dietary intake.

Beware of the Phantom Fat

You won't find partially hydrogenated vegetable oils listed on most food labels, but these manufactured oils are considered by many nutritionists to be hazardous to human health. Also known as *trans fatty acids*, these oils are manufactured by hydrogenating polyunsaturated oils so that they acquire many of the properties of saturated fat.

Identified by scores of studies as a primary cause of heart disease, trans fatty acids abound in margarine and vegetable shortening. This undesirable fat also finds its way into a huge variety of baked goods and processed foods like pie crusts and potato chips. Trans fatty acids are more stable than polyunsaturated oils so they can be used repeatedly for frying in restaurants. Fried chicken and seafood are often loaded with these free radical promoters.

Though they are named in lists of ingredients, the actual amount of trans fatty acid in any food is difficult to estimate. At some future date, food labels may be required to list their weight and daily value. Meanwhile, they remain a phantom fat that could undermine your health and suppress your immunity.

Fat substitutes, first introduced in 1996, may prove to be another hazard to your health and immunity. One leading brand is reported to inhibit absorption of carotenoids, a leading cancer-fighting chemical in plant foods. Watch out for these threatening fat substitutes in potato and tortilla chips and other snack foods. As for using them yourself, leave

201

them on the supermarket shelf and use olive or canola oil instead.

More Phantom Fats to Watch Out For

Trans fatty acids are not the only fats left out of food labels. The USDA defines "lean" meat as having no more than 10 percent fat by weight. But it has exempted ground beef. So "lean" ground beef can consist of as much as 22.5 percent fat by weight. And there's no way you can slice the fat off ground beef.

Other food label terminology can also be misleading. "Low fat" on a label means that the food contains no more than 3 grams of fat per serving. "Low calorie" on food labels indicates 40 calories or less per serving, and "light" means that either the fat content or the fat calories of the original food have been cut in half. For these terms to have any real meaning, you must first check the serving size. Is it one cup, half a cup or half a muffin? As time goes on, food label terminology could conceivably change, but as of the writing of this book, all these food traps still existed.

You may also be surprised by the relatively high-fat content of supposedly low-fat milk and other dairy products. In 2 percent milk, for example, 35 percent of the calories are from fat, with 5 grams of fat per serving. Meanwhile 1 percent milk still gets 18 to 23 percent of calories from fat. It's far safer to switch to nonfat dairy products like skim milk, powdered nonfat milk or skim buttermilk or to use nonfat cottage cheese, sour cream or plain nonfat yogurt. Fruit-flavored yogurts are also best avoided, as is ice cream made from whole milk and frozen yogurt look-alikes that are often loaded with sugar and fat.

It's worth noting, too, that nonfat dairy products still have the same content of animal protein as their high-fat counterparts. Anyone wanting to eliminate animal protein should certainly consider cutting back on dairy products, both nonfat and those with a higher fat content.

The Center for Science in the Public Interest has exposed most of the phantom fats in our foods. Their comments on chicken are worth heeding: "Chicken is not just chicken," they recently announced. "Four ounces of chicken breast have 4 grams of fat, while the drumstick has 6 grams and the thigh has 12 grams. And if you don't take the skin off, the fat doubles. Turkey breast has half the saturated fat of chicken breast. And no matter what the labels lead you to believe, 'lean' ground beef is virtually nonexistent."

Eat Enough Protein, But No More

A deficiency of protein can damage or even destroy the immune system. However, the average American consumes 160 percent of the RDA for protein and that extra 60 percent—which almost invariably consists of animal protein—is believed to fuel the growth of malignant tumors. Protein from plant foods does not appear to fuel cancer growth to the same extent.

Anyone who consumes 2,000 calories of food per day is unlikely to be deficient in protein. Yet studies have found that 50 percent of elderly men and women are protein deficient and their immune systems may be suppressed as a result. An older person weighing around 150 pounds is advised to eat about 2.5 ounces of protein per day. The problem is that too many older people eat diets that are marginally low in most nutrients. In just two months, that can cause a loss of 8 percent of body muscle and a reduced level of antibody production.

For most Americans, though, the problem is eating too much protein. An excess of protein may overburden the kidneys, and it has been linked to cancer of the colon, esophagus, lung, rectum and stomach.

A few years ago, during the China Health Study which analyzed the eating habits and diseases of the last surviving pockets of people in rural China who were still eating the diet of their ancestors, Dr. T. Colin Campbell and Dr. Chen Junschui discovered dramatic, statistically significant data in favor of obtaining protein from plant instead of animal foods.

Since a high cholesterol level results from eating a diet high in animal fat and protein, the doctors examined the cholesterol levels of people in various hospitals in rural China. They found that the people in the hospital with the highest serum cholesterol levels had a mortality rate from esophageal cancer 473 times higher than that in hospitals with the lowest cholesterol levels.

The authors concluded that the Chinese who consumed the most animal protein had the highest mortality from cancers of the stomach and esophagus and a significently greater incidence of cancers of the colon, lung and rectum, plus more leukemia than those who ate the least animal protein. The higher the cholesterol level, the greater the death rate from these types of cancer. One possible explanation is that a high-protein diet (that is, a diet high in meat and animal foods) increases the risk of these cancers, because people who eat large quantities of flesh foods have less room in their stomachs for vegetables, fruits and whole grains.

Eating adequate amounts of whole grains and beans each day ensures just about the right intake of whole protein without increasing the risk of cancer and heart diseases by eating flesh foods. Note, too, that adequate intake of vitamin C (preferably from fruit) is essential for the efficient synthesis of protein from plant sources.

Seven More Ways to Help Supercharge Your Immunity

Finally, here are seven ways to help supercharge your immunity by eating lean.

Tip 1. While cooking, you can eliminate from one-half to two-thirds the fat in most recipes without noticing the difference. For example, in recipes for muffins and other baked goods, substitute applesauce for 100 percent of the shortening. That also works for just about everything except cookies.

Tip 2. When shopping, avoid buying convenience foods such as the processed, manufactured, canned, packaged or prepared foods that line supermarket shelves. Replace them with real foods: fresh fruits, vegetables, whole grains, legumes, nuts and seeds, the same foods on which our ancestors thrived for millions of years. Half the so-called "food" eaten in America is embalmed, mass-produced convenience food loaded with fat and salt and ready to pop into the microwave or oven.

Another priceless shopping tip is to avoid the meat, deli and dairy sections in your supermarket and to zero in on the produce section. If you must buy meat, tenderloin, round or flank cuts of beef are lowest in fat. Also low are range-bred low-fat beef, wild game and sliced turkey or chicken breast. But they're all still high in animal protein, which some studies indicate may promote the growth of malignant tumors.

205

Before cooking, cut away all visible fat and remove all poultry skin. Your total daily intake from all flesh foods combined should never exceed 3.5 ounces—equivalent in size to a pack of playing cards.

However, it's a far better idea to replace all meat and poultry with plant-based meat substitutes such as tempeh, plain tofu, tofu hot dogs or soy- or grain-based hamburger. Soy products do contain monounsaturated fat, but it's far less harmful than the saturated fat which abounds in meat. Soy foods also contain phytomins believed to help prevent prostate and certain other cancers.

Tip 3. You can break an addiction to fat or sugar by eating only foods that grow on plants. To begin, make your first course at each meal exclusively plant-based foods. Start each meal with a green vegetable salad with nonfat dressing, a medium-sized bowl of vegetable soup or a bowl of whole wheat pasta. By the time you're ready for the high-fat, meat-centered main course, you'll find that much of your craving for meat and fat has evaporated.

Another effective way to dampen your desire for fat and meat is to drink 64 ounces of liquids such as water, skim milk, a sports drink, black, green or herbal tea or low-cal fruit juices each day. Sip 2 to 3 ounces at a time throughout the day.

Tip 4. Bake, broil, boil, steam, poach, stir-fry and saute but never, ever fry anything or eat any food that has been fried. Frying is a guaranteed way to transform a healthy food into a fat-laden promoter of free radicals, cancer and heart disease.

Watch, too, for fried vegetables. Broccoli, carrots, eggplant or spinach are all virtually fat-free. But they act as sponges when fried. A single serving can sop up 3 teaspoons of fat, equivalent to adding 135 calories, all from fat. Instead, stir-

206

fry these and other vegetables or saute them using a nonstick spray or defatted broth. And never forget that *all* cooking oils are 100 percent fat.

Tip 6. The earlier in the day a food is eaten, the less likely it is to end up as body fat. So make breakfast the largest meal of the day. Lunch should be more moderate in size, followed by a relatively light dinner. At all costs, don't skip breakfast. A Danish and coffee won't do either. Personally, I eat a 100 percent whole wheat cereal such as oatmeal or shredded wheat (my cereal usually totals two to three servings) and four fresh fruits such as a apple, banana, kiwi fruit, or pear and a large slice of cantaloupe—a total of six or more servings of plant-based foods—topped by a dollop of plain nonfat yogurt.

Tip 7. If you eat two or more servings each day of any of the foods on the following list, you are not eating a low-fat diet. Directly or indirectly, these foods assault the immune system, and they are also a major cause of heart disease, cancer, obesity and other degenerative diseases. Foods to avoid include, bacon, butter, cakes, cheese, cheesecake, cookies, croissants, dairy products except nonfat, eggs, fatty cuts of meat, French fries, all fried foods, ground beef, hamburgers, hot dogs, luncheon meats, margarine, muffins, pastries especially Danish, pecan rolls, pies, pizza made with cheese, potato chips, premium ice cream, red meat, ribs, salad dressings except nonfat, sausage and scones.

Is There Really an Obesity Gene?

Working in the National Institutes of Health respiratory chamber research project in Phoenix, scientists traced exactly what happens to fat when it's eaten. They found that

207

humans rarely turn carbohydrates into fat. Eating fat is what makes people fat.

They also discovered that overweight people are poor fat burners. They cannot handle foods containing fat. Average Americans get 34 percent of their calories from fat. But expert sources like the Framingham Heart Study and the prestigious National Research Council have recommended 15 percent as more appropriate.

Most health advisory agencies still recommend 30 percent or less because they feel that most Americans would not tolerate any lower percentage. But few of us notice that the recommended amount is 30 percent "or less." And less is obviously better.

Fat people do have a fat-burning impairment. It's called sedentary living. But this doesn't have to continue. For instance, the Pima Indians who live along the Mexican border in Arizona have a genuine inherited tendency to store fat. Three out of four tribal members are obese. Yet the genetically identical Pima Indians who live a few miles away in Mexico weigh, on average, 50 pounds less. The explanation: The Mexican Indian men spend 40 hours a week or more toiling in the fields while the women expend 60 hours on active house and garden work. The Mexican Pimas also eat a predominently complex carbohydrate diet based on beans, corn and vegetables with only 23 percent of their calories derived from fat.

In Arizona, where machines do all the work and the fat intake is much higher, the fat-burning impairment leads to obesity. But as the Mexican Pimas have demonstrated, it doesn't have to. Regardless of whether we have a fat-burning impairment or not, we can definitely beat it by making wise health choices and then exerting our muscles and minds to do what it takes to succeed.

IMMUNE BOOSTER #7: Don't Let Food-Borne Infections Overload Your Immunity

An important step in preventing immune-system overload is to protect our immune systems from having to fight off food-borne infections. According to the Center for Science in the Public Interest and other food safety organizations, America's meat, poultry, eggs and shellfish are often contaminated with bacteria, some of which can cause serious illness or possibly death.

Not surprisingly, perhaps, most of the foods that are contaminated are the same gremlin foods that overload the immune system in other ways. All these health-robbing foods are identified and listed in IB #3, together with an explanation of how they overload the immune system by promoting the development of free radicals, cancer and degenerative diseases.

But while degenerative diseases take years or decades to appear, most food-borne diseases make their presence known within hours or a day at the most. And while not all food-borne diseases are serious, many can cause nausea, vomiting, diarrhea and dehydration. Destroying these food-borne bacteria places an excessive load on the immune system that could temporarily suppress it. Whenever the body is unprotected by a powerful immune system, a malignant tumor could develop.

Food-Borne Interlopers That Could Compromise Immunity

Staphylococcal food poisoning is the most common food-borne disease. It causes diarrhea and intestinal distress but

209

usually clears up in 24 hours. Half of us carry staphylococcus bacteria on our hands and the disease is commonly transmitted by food handlers.

Salmonella bacteria is common in the bodies of farm animals and poultry and is not killed by freezing. Diarrhea is the principal symptom of salmonellosis. Most cases are mild, but it can become serious and require emergency medical treatment.

Cyclospora is a parasite that causes severe stomach cramps and vomiting. Among more severe food-borne diseases are bacillic and amebic dysentery and cholera, all of which are common in less developed countries.

If diarrhea, vomiting and other symptoms do not clear up in 2 to 3 days, you should see a doctor. Severe, watery diarrhea is particularly dangerous, and if left untreated, it may lead to prostration, collapse or even meningitis.

Where Risk of Infection Is Greatest

Certainly, the outer skin of some fruits and vegetables may harbor salmonella or cyclospora. But the risk of food-borne infection is far greater in meat, poultry, eggs and shellfish.

Due to their greater surface area, ground beef and hamburger are far more perishable and more likely to cause food poisoning than other meats. They are often exposed to bacteria during grinding. Twenty-five percent of ground beef in the United States is currently estimated to carry the bacteria *E.coli 0157:H7*, a microbe that may cause kidney failure and related disorders in people with suppressed or immature immune systems, particularly children under 10 and older people.

Heat kills bacteria, but chicken and ground meat are often

undercooked. Failure to completely thaw frozen meat before cooking is a common cause of undercooking. Overcooking or barbecuing may also char flesh foods, forming potentially carcinogenic burned areas. If not well-cooked, chicken and other poultry are a frequent source of infectious diseases such as salmonella and campylobacter.

Raw shellfish can contain infectious microbes from human sewage. Each year, approximately 100,000 Americans become sick eating raw shellfish. Few of us realize that when we eat shellfish, we consume the organism's entire digestive system, including its feces.

Raw eggs, such as those used to make batter, may also contain salmonella. Unless thoroughly cooked, any egg may cause salmonella poisoning; the symptoms range from intestinal discomfort, diarrhea and vomiting to severe illness or possibly death.

Kitchen sponges and dishrags are often contaminated with bacteria from meat, poultry, eggs or shellfish and can spread infectious microbes all over the kitchen. Mouldy bread, cheeses and peanuts, and any kind of raw fish or seafood, are other common sources of food poisoning.

New Food-Borne Infections May Be Incurable

Since the 104th Congress weakened food safety laws to allow food manufacturers to make greater profits, new and often incurable forms of food-borne diseases have begun to appear. Widespread use of antibiotics in animal and poultry feed has enabled bacteria to develop resistance to these drugs and to flourish more than ever. When they appear in humans, these new bacteria strains are often incurable.

Obviously, food-borne infections of this caliber can seri-

211

ously overload the immune system, allowing cancer cells to escape detection and to clone into a tumor. Equally obvious, the best way to avoid a food-borne infection is to avoid eating meat, poultry, eggs and shellfish. These and other health-robbing foods are all listed in IB #3: Cut Back on Foods That Cripple Your Immune System.

Whether or not you continue to eat counterproductive foods, here is what you need to know to prevent overloading your immune system with food-borne infections. These precautions can also help you avoid the extremely unpleasant and sometimes dangerous symptoms that these infections cause.

Assume That All Eggs and Flesh Foods Are Contaminated

Several health-advisory agencies have advised Americans to assume that all eggs, raw meat, poultry and shellfish are contaminated. When eating out, always order meat and poultry well-done, especially hamburgers and ground beef. Never eat any meat or poultry that is pink on the inside or cooked "rare."

Eggs

Salmonella is so widespread in the United States that many eggs are infected while developing inside hens, and then the bacteria multiplies rapidly during storage and shipment. Never eat raw or partially cooked eggs, and don't remove eggs from the stove while they are still runny. Eggs are safe to eat only when the whites are completely firm and the yolk has thickened. Several public health authorities asked me to strongly emphasize that *all* eggs are a major source of salmonella and *must be cooked thoroughly.*

Meat and Poultry

According to Tufts University researchers, as much as 25 percent of ground beef sold in American supermarkets may contain bacteria capable of causing salmonellosis and related disorders. Salmonella can be caused by 50 different varieties of *E. coli* bacteria, each of which produces a toxin called *shiga.* The immune system is able to identify the antigen of these bacteria as unfriendly while permitting billions of other, friendly varieties of *E. coli* to thrive in our colons.

When raw beef is ground into hamburger, bacteria on the surface of the meat is churned into the interior. Grinding also increases the surface area of meat many times over. The result is that bacteria can easily survive and infect ground beef (or any other ground meat, including mincemeat and pork). Grinding may also spread bacteria from the meat of one animal to another.

To prevent infection, first be sure that any frozen flesh food has completely thawed all the way through. The safest way to cook it then is by microwaving. Heat it for 30 to 90 seconds on "high," or until the juices begin to flow. Then pour off the juices and begin cooking.

To avoid exposing other foods to shiga toxins when shopping, have meat, poultry, eggs, fish and seafood bagged in a completely separate plastic bag that does not contain, nor is in contact with, any other foods. Fruits and vegetables are often contaminated by juices from raw flesh foods while inside shopping bags in hot weather (or inside warm cars at any time). The same precautions should be taken in the refrigerator. Keep flesh foods at the bottom where juices cannot drip onto other foods.

213

Be careful not to place cooked meats, poultry or any other foods on a plate containing raw juices from flesh foods. Clean all poultry thoroughly before cooking and cook well. Never eat "pink" chicken. And never drink raw milk.

Roughly 25 percent of all chicken currently sold in the United States is contaminated with salmonella and up to 90 percent are contaminated with campylobacter. In the future, the FDA may be able to reduce these rates somewhat by improving hygiene in poultry processing plants.

Shellfish and Fish

Shellfish such as clams, mussels and oysters each filter about 2.5 gallons of seawater through their bodies each hour, straining out and retaining everything in it, including microbes and human sewage. Moreover, just about all shellfish taken from Gulf of Mexico waters between May and November are infected with *Vibrio vunificus*, a bacteria that can prove fatal to humans if eaten raw. As with all other flesh foods and eggs, the golden rule is to always eat fish and seafood well-cooked.

Fruits and Vegetables

Overripe bananas, cantaloupe, sprouts, tomatoes and watermelon are inviting cultures for salmonella, while strawberries and other berries that cannot be peeled may harbor the parasite *cyclospora*. Tainted cabbage may be infected with listeria and mushrooms with campylobacter. Wherever possible, all other fruits and vegetables should be scrubbed with clean water before eating. (However, don't wash with water, such as tapwater in Mexico, if you think it might be contaminated.)

214

Provided you do the peeling yourself, most peelable fruits and vegetables are safe to eat, even in underdeveloped countries. Traces of pesticide can be removed by rinsing the fruit or vegetable in a pint of warm water into which a few drops of dish soap have been dissolved; be sure to rinse thoroughly afterward.

The deadly bacteria *E. coli 0157:57* is appearing in produce imported from Third World countries that have less rigorous sanitation standards than ours. During the winter, 70 percent of fruits and vegetables may be imported from these countries. Buyer beware.

I suggest never eating sprouts unless they are thoroughly crisp and fresh. From personal observation, I estimate that 50 percent of those served in restaurants are spoiled. In any case, sprouts have scored so low in recent nutrient analysis tests that they are no longer regarded as the wonder foods we once thought.

Kitchen Sponges and Utensils

In any kitchen where uncooked meat, poultry, eggs and seafood have been handled, kitchen sponges and dishrags— together with all boards, utensils and plates that have been in contact with these foods—are likely to be contaminated. Once the foods are in the oven, all should be thoroughly washed in an antibacterial cleanser. Then, after washing your hands in hot, soapy water, clean up any remaining juices or traces with paper towels and discard. Because shiga-producing bacteria multiply rapidly if left overnight, be sure to thoroughly clean everything which has been in contact with raw flesh foods or eggs before touching anything else.

215

CHAPTER SIX

The Physical Approach: Using the Body to Revitalize Your Immunity

O ur immune system is a mirror of our physical appearance and of how good we look and feel. If we're overweight and out-of-shape, our self-esteem falters and we feel depressed. When this happens, our immuno-competence plummets right along with the way we feel about ourselves.

But we can make the opposite happen.

As we restore the appearance of our body through exercise, our self-esteem soars, our mood becomes elevated and our immuno-competence regains much of its original youthful vigor.

216

Exercise is one of the quickest and best ways to supercharge your immunity and restore its youthful vitality. By exercising and improving the way you look and feel, your immune system will immediately mirror your new, improved appearance and the new, optimistic way you feel about yourself. And your immuno-competence will soar.

Nothing Ages Us Faster Than Being Overweight

Not only does excess poundage make us look and feel older, but it biologically speeds up the aging of every part of the body, including the immune system. A man or woman who has gained 10 to 15 pounds since age 21, and whose waistline has increased more than 2 to 3 inches, has a significantly higher risk of immuno-suppression, as well as cancer and infectious diseases, than a person with a BMI of under 25. Yet two-thirds of Americans are overweight and by age 65, the average sedentary man or woman has lost 35 percent of lung capacity and one-third of the heart's capacity to pump blood.

In both men and women who fail to exercise, the heart muscle weakens and the heart becomes smaller. Arteries harden, become partially blocked and lose their flexibility. Together with the rest of the body, the immune system enters into a state of rapid aging and decline.

But HNRC researchers discovered, this litany of decay is not inevitable. Provided no actual damage has occurred to the cardiovascular and other systems, a corpulent body can be restored to health. Through a gradually increasing program of daily exercise, it is usually possible to restore our heart, lungs, arteries and immune system to a much more youthful and healthy condition.

Through a combination of aerobic and strength-building

exercise practiced daily, these amazing benefits can occur at almost any age and regardless of how long a person has been sedentary. Providing we keep exercising and eating a lean diet, we can win back a strong heart, healthy lungs and clear arteries and we can restore to our immune system much of the vigor it had years ago. When this happens, little or no age-related damage need occur either in our bodies or in our immune systems until quite late in life.

Being Unfit Is As Dangerous As Smoking

Recent studies have clearly demonstrated that physical in-activity is a well-defined major risk factor for impaired im-munity as well as overall health. For instance, a 1996 study at the Cooper Institute for Aerobic Research in Dallas concluded that a low level of fitness is as dangerous to health as smoking two packs of cigarettes per day. The study, known as the Aerobics Center Longitudinal Study, found that a low level of physical activity was a strong predictor of death from all causes. The study also demonstrated that men or women with another health risk were less likely to die if they exercised than was a healthy person who did not exercise. For example, an overweight person who is physically fit has a higher level of wellness than a slender person who is unfit.

Literally hundreds of well-documented studies have clearly shown that regular exercise, combined with a lean diet, prevents heart disease, stroke, hypertension, diabetes and most other chronic diseases.

But until recently, the link between exercise and diet, on the one hand, and cancer prevention, on the other, was not as well known. This knowledge is particularly important for strengthening the immunity because cancer cells or tumors can overburden and weaken the immune system.

218

Derail Cancer with Exercise

Another Cooper Institute survey of 12,975 men with a starting age of 44 found that between 1970 and 1989, those who did the most aerobic exercise had the lowest prostate cancer rates. Men who performed a moderate level of rhythmic exercise (burning 2,000 to 3,000 calories a week) reduced their prostate cancer risk by 25 percent. But those who did a high level of aerobic exercise (3,000 to 4,000 calories per week) reduced their risk by 70 percent. Though 3,000 to 4,000 calories may sound like a lot, it's equivalent to walking only 2 miles per day at a brisk 4 mph.

Similar studies have shown the same results, leading researchers to conclude that exercise reduces levels of the male hormone testosterone. In animal studies, rodents with the lowest testosterone levels have always had the lowest prostate cancer risks.

Several other studies show that women who perform a total of 4 hours of rhythmic exercise each week reduce their risk of breast cancer by 50 to 60 percent. Those who have exercised regularly since their teens had the lowest risk, indicating that a life-long pattern of exercise since childhood may be crucial to cancer prevention. Other studies show that both men and women with physically active jobs are 60 percent less likely to develop colon cancer.

Evidence is overwhelming that regular exercise dramatically reduces risk of breast, colorectal and prostate cancer as well as cancer of the cervix, ovaries, uterus and vagina. Much of the reduced risk is believed due to a lower level of sex hormones in men and women who exercise daily at a fairly vigorous level.

Putting it all together, when combined with a lean diet, regular daily exercise:

- Benefits every cell and organ in the body, especially the immune system.
- Significantly reduces risk of most cancers, particularly those that are hormone-related.
- Stimulates the bowels to empty more rapidly and keeps the colon clear of cancer-causing wastes. Exercise is as effective as a high-fiber diet in preventing colorectal cancer.
- Prevents and reduces obesity, a condition which suppresses the immune system on several different levels.
- Elevates mood, one of the strongest Immune Boosters in existance.
- Retards aging of the entire body, including aging of immune cells. Therefore the immune system remains more vigorous and youthful.

The Lethal Trap of Sedentary Living

Despite these findings, a recent Centers for Disease Control survey reports that 60 percent of U.S. adults do not perform sufficient exercise to benefit health and 25 percent are totally inactive. The report also found that inactivity increases with age, is more common among older women than older men and is most common among both sexes of lower socioeconomic backgrounds.

As sedentary people lose their strength, stamina and quality of life, they become stiffer, develop arthritis and put on weight. Soon, their immunity heads south and they become prey to a melancholy list of infections and diseases.

If you hope to supercharge your immunity, you cannot allow yourself to fall into the trap of sedentary living. To rejuvenate your immune system, and to keep it in top condition, regular daily exercise is a must, not an option.

220

Once you begin to exercise, it's important to never miss a session. Once you give in or give up, your immunity will head downhill once more. So set aside an exercise period each day and don't allow anything to derail your plans. For this reason, many people exercise first thing in the morning before anything can interfere.

Personally, I never allow lack of equipment or the inability to go outdoors to prevent me from exercising. Scores of stretching, calisthenics and isometric exercises can be done on the living room floor or in a motel room. You can then run in place without needing anything in the way of equipment.

Exercising with a friend or a group may be more fun, but don't miss a session because you may have to work out by yourself. Most health clubs, spas, gyms, pools or senior centers offer group exercise classes at nominal cost. With or without a companion, you can still make exercise your top priority—as essential as sleeping or eating and not the last thing on your list.

Why We Have No Time for Exercise

When people tell me they have no time for exercise, I ask how many hours a day they spend watching TV. Surveys show that most Americans spend between 2.5 and 4 hours daily glued to the tube. Even if it were only two hours, that totals 14 hours a week—or an entire waking day—spent in a stupor watching a babbling video screen.

To liberate yourself from this giant thief of time, learn to recognize television for what it really is—an uninvited intrusion of advertisers into the privacy of your home. Just about all commercial TV exposes you to advertising by luring you to watch shows that all too often are violent and raunchy.

Even news programs are a form of entertainment built around news items for which the studio has the most graphic footage or which it considers most entertaining. If you want really informative news, you can read it on the Internet, updated every 15 minutes and featuring only the most newsworthy items, rather than those that use the best visual entertainment to draw viewers to watch the ads.

To free yourself from the shackles of TV, watch only shows that make you laugh and you will surely have ample time for exercise. Some cable stations also present occasional exercise programs. I limit TV watching only to programs that are truly inspiring or to documentaries about health, fitness and adventure travel—most of which are on public television.

You can probably free up another 30 to 45 minutes each day by cutting out afterwork social or family get-togethers such as dinners, coffees, drinks or barbecues. Next to TV, social chatting on the phone is one of the greatest time-wasters in modern living. And how much time do you spend reading nonessential stories in the newspaper each day? You might also save valuable time on weekends by cutting back on housekeeping chores, vacuuming the rug only twice a month instead of once a week, for instance.

If activities like these are important to you, by all means continue them. But for many of us, they're simply time-consuming intrusions that destroy our leisure and prevent us from exercising.

Watching Sports Events May Increase Cancer Risk

Since cancer can exert an overload situation on the immune system, it's interesting to learn that watching sports on

TV can possibly increase the risk of a hormone-related cancer. When Dr. James Dabb of Georgia State University collected testosterone samples from the saliva of male spectators who had just watched a soccer match between Italy and Brazil, he found that supporters of the winning team experienced a rise in testosterone levels of 27 percent, while supporters of the losing side experienced a testosterone drop of an equal amount.

Results are too preliminary to suggest that watching ball games on TV increases the risk of cancer. Yet the male hormone testosterone is the driving force behind the growth of prostate tumors.

A WHOLE-PERSON EXERCISE PROGRAM TO HELP BOOST IMMUNITY

For best results, I recommend doing an aerobic workout one day followed by a strength-training workout the next for a total of six days each week.

- Aerobics is any form of brisk, rhythmic exercise such as walking, swimming or bicycling that employs the body's large muscle groups in continuous, unbroken movement sufficiently vigorous to raise heartbeat and breathing rates and oxygen uptake. Aerobics restores tone to flabby muscles and helps burn off excess weight. IB #8 describes aerobic exercise and how to get started.
- Strength-training exercise increases the body's lean muscle mass, raises metabolism and gradually burns off excess weight. Strength-training exercise rapidly rebuilds atrophied muscles and sculpts the body back into shape.

223

Doing so creates a tremendous boost in self-esteem that is immediately mirrored in the immune system. IB #9 describes strength-training exercise and how to get started.

The Power of Body, Mind and Nutrition Working Together

I'd like to emphasize that exercise is far more likely to supercharge the immune system when it is part of a comprehensive whole-person approach. Thus I recommend that you make it a part of IB #5: The 8-Step Weight Loss and Immune-Boosting Program. While exercise is the core of this program, it also guides you toward adopting IB #4: The One Diet That Does It All, plus the other nutritional Immune Boosters #2, #3 and #6.

You are also advised to add visualization, a powerful mind technique described in IB #17. Working through subtle mechanisms in the brain, visualization can also empower you to begin exercising and to stay with it. Visualization also allows you to practice exercise movements—such as swimming strokes or strength-training techniques—while relaxing or lying in bed. A comprehensive whole-person approach like this invariably produces results that are superior to using exercise alone.

You're Never Too Old to Begin

Provided you have no medical or orthopedic problem, few men or women are too old to benefit from an exercise program. Several years ago, for example, Dr. Maria Fiatarone enrolled 63 women and 37 men, all between the ages of 72 and 98, into a strength-building study at Boston's Hebrew Rehab Center for the Aged. The average age was 87 and one-third were over 90.

One-third of participants worked out regularly on strength-training machines, one-third took nutritional supplements and one-third did nothing. A few weeks later, everyone in the strength-training group had increased their muscle size and strength, their walking speed and their stair-climbing ability. They also displayed powerful psychological benefits including an enhanced self-image, confidence, optimism and a greatly improved quality of life—all factors that boost immuno-competence. Nutritional supplements alone produced no increase in strength or mobility.

This, and several similar studies, have proven conclusively that regardless of age or how atrophied a person's muscles may be, both strength and muscle mass, as well as cardiovascular health and aerobic ability, can all be improved by daily exercise. *Any such improvement immediately triggers a corresponding improvement in immuno-competence.*

Read This Caveat Before You Start Exercising

Most health advisory agencies agree that, for the average person, the risk of *not* exercising far outweighs any risk of a gradually increasing program of daily exercise. Most healthy men or women aged 35 or younger can safely begin a daily walking program at a moderate pace. As your fitness improves, you can gradually walk a little farther and faster each day. Even so, you are cautioned never to exceed your capacity. Avoid becoming tired or fatigued and never push yourself to the limit—at least, not until you have become exceptionally well-conditioned (see IB #10).

If you are over 35 and have any of the following symptoms

225

or conditions, you should see a doctor before you begin to exercise:

You consume more than two alcoholic drinks a day or are a steady smoker.

You suffer from a chronic disease or dysfunction such as heart disease, hypertension, angina, claudication, stroke, cancer, renal disease or any pulmonary disease.

You are unable to walk a mile in 17.5 minutes.

You are on any medication, especially beta-blockers.

You experience chest pain, dizziness or shortness of breath with or without exertion.

You have diabetes or have cuts, wounds and burns on your feet that don't heal or are slow to heal.

You have lost weight during the past six months without trying.

You experience fast or irregular heartbeats or very slow beats after exertion.

You have osteoporosis, have suffered an injury in hip, knee, spine, wrist or other joint, have arthritis or have had a fall.

You have any orthopedic or cardiovascular problem;

You are more than 20 pounds overweight.

If you have one or more of these conditions, see a doctor regardless of your age. The older and heavier you are, the more vital it is to see a doctor before exercising. Again, if you are recovering from an injury, have any form of disability or have had joint surgery or a joint replacement, your doctor or a physical therapist should plan your exercise workout.

A final caution: Not all doctors believe in exercise. To avoid being given biased advice by a doctor who may be unfamiliar with the benefits of exercise, consult only a physician who is obviously lean and fit and who is known to favor therapeutic exercise.

Although I've emphasized exercise in this introduction, it in no way diminishes the importance of the other physical Immune Boosters in this chapter. Equally important are the many things you can do to avoid being infected by viruses or bacteria, all described in IB #11. And a few hours of unprotected solar exposure can send your immunity plunging for two weeks at a time (see IB #12). In addition, millions of Americans under 45 suffer from self-inflicted sleep deprivation, one of the most powerful and widespread immunosuppressors (see IB #13).

IMMUNE BOOSTER #8: Unlock Your Immune Power with Aerobic Exercise

---

When Bill was 60 years old, his cardiologist diagnosed severe blockage of the coronary arteries while his urologist diagnosed stage B prostate cancer. The cancer was confirmed by ultrasound and a biopsy. Tests also showed that his immune system was suppressed.

Bill's cardiologist recommended a bypass operation. But Bill was terrified of hospitals and surgery. Instead, he chose to enroll at a live-in cardiac rehabilitation center that specialized in reversing coronary artery disease using diet and exercise.

Once at the center, Bill quickly learned that 80 percent

227

of bypass operations were really unnecessary and that they were done primarily for economic reasons and because most men and women are unwilling to make the required lifestyle changes. While Bill's rehabilitation might take several weeks or months, he would have to pay the cost himself. By comparison, a bypass operation would be fully covered by his insurance and he could return to work in a few weeks.

More importantly, perhaps, since bypass operations are almost universally recommended by all doctors in the region where Bill lived, no physician dared to recommend any non-medical alternative. No one diagnosed with heart disease was ever told that going to a rehabilitation center was one of his or her options. Should a physician do so, and a patient died, the physician could be sued for failing to adhere to the standard medical procedures practiced in that region.

Bill also learned that three times as many bypass operations are done per capita in some parts of the country than in others, with no difference in quality of life or life expectancy.

Medical Treatment May Not Always Be in the Patient's Best Interests

Learning that medical advice and treatment are often dictated by finances and politics, rather than by what is in the patient's best interests, merely reinforced Bill's determination to prove to his doctor that heart disease *could* be reversed without surgery or drugs. Bill was put on a diet almost identical to that described in IB #4: The One Diet That Does It All. Simultaneously, he began a structured program of gradually increasing daily walks.

At first, Bill could walk only 200 yards before experiencing chest pains. But, under supervision, he continued to walk several times each day. Each time he was able to walk a little farther and faster before his angina pain began.

Then, almost miraculously, on the tenth day, his chest pains disappeared. Bill was able to walk a mile at a time. Already his Body Mass Index, which had been 28, had dropped to 27 and was headed steadily down.

Once he was able to walk briskly for 35 minutes each morning, Bill's endorphin effect kicked in and he felt terrific and optimistic for the rest of the day. This success triggered his enabling effect. In turn, this boosted his placebo effect. Translated, this meant that Bill had suddenly developed an awesome ability to tap into his healing-regeneration system.

Five weeks later, Bill's Body Mass Index had dropped to a healthy 24 and his doctors pronounced him free from all danger of a heart attack. He was sent home with strict instructions to stay on his diet and to continue to exercise daily for the rest of his life.

The Immune System Seems to Thrive on Exercise and a Lean Diet

But Bill's greatest surprise came when he visited his urologist.

"I've never seen anything quite like this," the urologist exclaimed, "but your PSA level has dropped by 25 percent and your prostate tumor seems to have actually shrunk."

The only explanation the urologist could give was that the vigor of Bill's immune system had somehow become supercharged. When that happened, the urologist surmised, his T-cells and macrophages must have attacked the prostate tumor and partially destroyed it.

229

"Whatever you're doing, keep it up," the urologist advised. "I suspect that your aerobic exercise, plus losing weight, plus your lean diet, plus your switch to an optimistic attitude all worked together to beef up your immunity."

Although Bill's tumor did not disappear entirely, it remained dormant and never grew larger. Of the various therapies he used, Bill believed that aerobic exercise was the underlying factor that triggered his recovery.

More Evidence That Exercise and Eating Lean Benefit Immunity

While this particular case history does not prove that aerobic exercise boosts immunity, a number of similar cases seem to suggest that it might. Rheumatoid arthritis is a disease caused when the immune system goes awry and attacks the lining of joints in the body. Scores of cases have been recorded in which men and women with both heart disease and rheumatoid arthritis were sent to rehabilitation centers to recover from their heart disease. As they walked each day and ate a lean diet, their arteries began to open up and their heart disease gradually faded. At the same time, many saw their rheumatoid arthritis disappear as well. And for as long as they stayed with the lean diet and the aerobic exercise, they remained free of both heart disease *and* rheumatoid arthritis. Somehow the combination of lean diet and aerobic exercise restored the balance of their immune systems so that their immune cells ceased to attack tissue in their own bodies.

Without exception every health advisory agency recommends exercising aerobically at least three times each week.

That's because aerobic exercise benefits every cell, organ and system in the body, including the immune system.

Several surveys have shown that a brisk 35-minute walk each day could prevent or reverse half of all the diseases and dysfunctions from which Americans suffer and could save billions of dollars annually on surgery and drugs.

Starting an Aerobic Workout

Aerobic exercise is any brisk, rhythmic movement of the large muscles of the arms and legs sufficiently vigorous to raise your heart and breathing rates and to increase your oxygen uptake. As you walk, swim, bicycle or perform any similar aerobic exercise, you automatically inhale large amounts of oxygen that aerate the blood, which the heart then forcefully pumps through the arteries to energize the muscles. Increasing your ability to process oxygen in this way also increases your aerobic capacity.

Walking is the most readily available aerobic exercise, but any similar rhythmic workout can produce a dramatic increase in aerobic capacity within 2 to 3 months provided you exercise regularly three to four times each week.

To get started, simply begin walking at an easy pace, then gradually increase your speed and distance as your fitness improves. To provide real benefit, an aerobic exercise must be continuous. If you're going too fast and have to stop and rest, slow down to a pace you can maintain comfortably without stopping. That's one reason why stop-and-go exercises like walking a golf course or doubles tennis provide few, if any, aerobic benefits.

Most beginners start to walk at a relaxed pace of about 2.75 mph. Walking casually like this for, say, a 20-minute exercise period may prevent a heart attack, but it is seldom vigorous enough to provide any real aerobic benefit, burn surplus fat or revitalize your immune system.

So as soon as you can, increase your speed to a normal walking speed of 3 to 3.75 mph. Keep your arms loose and extended and swing them as you walk. Many beginners soon find they can walk a 17-minute mile. Soon afterward, they can walk 3 miles in 50 minutes. Walking this fast should raise your pulse rate to a level where "training effect" occurs. Training effect occurs when you walk fast enough to keep your pulse rate in your personal heart target zone.

How to Calculate Your Exercise Target Zone

Your personal target zone depends on your age. You can calculate it like this:

Step 1. Subtract your age from 220. The result is your maximum heart rate ("max") which you should never exceed. For a 60-year-old person, subtracting 60 from 220 leaves 160, the maximum number of heartbeats per minute for a 60-year-old.

Step 2. Your heart target zone lies between 70 and 85 percent of max. Seventy percent of 160 is 112, the lower limit; 85 percent of 160 is 136, the upper limit.

Thus the heart target zone for a 60-year-old person lies between 112 and 136 heartbeats per minute.

To revitalize your cardiovascular system, you need to exercise aerobically at a pace that elevates your pulse rate into your target zone and keeps it there for 30 to 50 minutes on three or more occasions each week. Once your heartbeat enters your target zone, the phenomenon called *training effect* occurs which challenges the body to maximize its aerobic capacity.

The Amazing Benefits of Training Effect

After working out in your target zone for a few weeks, training effect frequently produces an amazing increase in aerobic capacity and cardiovascular fitness. Often unexpectedly, exercisers find they can inhale large amounts of oxygen into their lungs while the heart is able to forcibly deliver large amounts of oxygen-rich blood to the body with every beat.

In response to training effect, the heart has learned to pump a much greater volume of blood with each beat. Most exercisers are suddenly endowed with almost tireless energy and with a youthful level of stamina and endurance. Both men and women find they can walk miles without feeling tired while their resting pulse rate drops to a healthy 60 to 65 beats per minute. In fact, the heart has responded so well to training effect that it now requires an increase in walking speed and distance before the pulse rate will enter the target zone at all.

To enter your target zone, you must now speed up your pulse and breathing rate. You do this by walking faster. For instance, most beginners can enter their target zone by increasing their walking speed by one-fourth. If you begin walking at a casual speed of 2.75 mph, accelerating your pace to 3.25 mph should elevate your heart rate into the lower levels of your target zone.

To do so, you'll probably have to swing your arms and take brisker, longer strides. Almost any reasonably healthy

233

person can enter the target zone for a minute or two. If you get out of breath, you are probably in your target zone. That's because the less fit you are, the less rapidly you need to walk to enter your zone.

As you become fitter and your heart pumps more blood with each beat, you must walk farther and faster to stay in your target zone. At first, you can probably stay in your zone for only 2 to 3 minutes. But as you continue to exercise aerobically, you will find yourself able to stay in your target zone for longer and longer periods of time.

Walking in Your Target Zone

It's important to grasp this principle. For example, walking 1 mile at 3.25 mph is sufficient to stimulate the hearts of most beginners to reach a pulse rate equivalent to at least 70 percent of max.

But after exercising aerobically for a few weeks, your conditioning should improve to where you can walk 1 mile at 3.25 mph easily and without much effort. Once you reach this level, walking at 3.25 mph is no longer sufficient to keep your heart in your target zone.

To reach 70 percent of max, you must now walk 2 miles at 3.25 mph, or 1 mile at 3.5 mph. As your conditioning improves, you must increase your pace and distance to remain in your target zone for the same length of time.

Eventually, of course, you'll reach a fitness plateau which will keep your heart in your target zone without further increases of distance or speed. For example, once you're able to walk briskly for 60 minutes, you should be able to stay in your target zone for 50 of those minutes. During these 50 minutes you should easily cover 3 miles.

234

At this point, your aerobic intensity should be in the 15 to 16 range (see the table with the Scale of Perceived Exertion below) and you will be in your target zone during most of your workout. As training effect occurs, you will experience a sudden huge boost in energy, stamina and aerobic capacity. Training effect *will* occur with any kind of aerobic exercise, whether it's walking, jogging, swimming, bicycling, rowing, cross-country skiing or whether you're replicating one of these activities on an exercise machine.

By then, walking at 4 mph should be relatively easy. With arms swinging, walking at this brisk pace becomes a whole body exercise that tones arm, leg and buttock muscles while trimming the waist and bolstering immunity. The benefits are even greater when you also eat lean (see IBs #3, #4, #5 and #6) and begin using psychological action-steps to boost your motivation and performance (see IB #17).

How to Tell When You're Exercising
in Your Target Zone

How can you tell while exercising whether your pulse is in your target zone? One way is to wear a heart monitor. Another is to stop and take your pulse for 10 seconds, then multiply the number of beats by six. However, the American College of Sports Medicine, along with most exercise physiologists, claim that sensing your exertion level by gut feeling is superior to any measurement based on pulse rate.

Depending on how hard or how easy your workout feels, the table below helps you make a fairly accurate estimate of whether you are in or out of your target zone.

Scale of Perceived Exertion

Exertion Level	Aerobic Intensity*	Percentage of Max
Maximum exertion	20	
Extremely hard	18-19	100
Very hard	16-17	80
Hard	14-15	70
Somewhat hard	12-13	60
Light	10-11	50
Very light	8-9	35
Extremely light	7	20
None	6	

*These numbers are not related to heartbeat but represent an arbitrary scale of exertion.

Let the Way You Feel Be Your Heart Monitor

During tests, people who rated their workout as "extremely hard" were usually exercising at max, "very hard" was equivalent to 80 percent of max, "hard" equalled 70 percent of max and "somewhat hard" indicated 60 percent of max. You should always stay below a feeling of "extremely hard," or at least enter it only for very brief periods and then only if you are in excellent condition.

To experience how it feels to be in your target zone, stop and take your pulse for 10 seconds while walking at various levels of exertion and after having walked various distances. Note how your breathing and exertion feel when walking at 60, 70 and 80 percent of max.

Here are other indicators: After walking 1 mile at a pace brisk enough to cause mild perspiration, you are probably exercising at around 65 percent of max. If at the same time you can carry on a conversation, you are probably not exceeding 70 to 75 percent of max.

Walking while in your target zone provides all the benefits

236

of jogging without the risk of injury that afflicts so many joggers. Once you're really fit, you can intensify your workout by walking briskly up and down hills.

Should you be unable to walk briskly enough to enter your target zone, consider walking for a longer distance at a more moderate pace. Known as long slow distance (LSD) training, any type of aerobic exercise performed at an easier pace can provide aerobic benefit by virtue of the longer time and distance covered. A long, moderately paced walk—or any other type of aerobic exercise—is particularly effective for burning body fat.

Can Aerobic Exercise Burn Off Body Fat?

When our metabolism is high, we burn body fat much more rapidly than when it is low. (Metabolism is explained in IB #6 together with instructions for calculating your personal nonresting metabolic rate.) A fairly intense aerobic workout can keep your nonresting metabolic rate elevated for several hours during and after an exercise period. The more intense the aerobic exercise, and the longer we do it, the higher our nonresting metabolic rate will rise and the longer it will remain elevated.

Intense exercise is the same as exercising in your target zone, and exercising in the zone burns several hundred calories per hour. For every 3,500 calories expended in aerobic exercise, 1 pound of body fat is burned. To lose 1 pound in 10 days, you have to expend 350 more calories per day in exercise than you consume in food. The table below gives the approximate number of calories burned per hour by a 150-pound person performing different types of aerobic exercise.

237

Calories Burned Per Hour by Aerobic Exercise

Rowing machine, moderate pace	325
Brisk walking at 4 mph	345
Square dancing	350
Bicycling at 12 mph	500
Swimming at 1 mph	535
Fast walking at 5 mph	550
Cross-country skiing	580
Rowing machine, vigorous pace	650
Vigorous stair climbing	675

According to the table, a 150-pound person who spends an hour a day square dancing or walking briskly at 4 mph, should easily knock a pound off his or her weight in 10 days. Or an hour a day of rowing, swimming, fast walking or stair climbing at a more vigorous pace burns off 1 pound of fat in only 7 days.

By comparison, 1 hour of strength-training exercise burns about 300 calories. By alternating an hour of vigorous aerobic exercise one day with an hour of strength-training exercise the next day, you could easily burn off 1 pound of fat every 10 days. And to lose stubborn fat, we ideally need both strength-training and aerobic workouts.

Interval Training Burns Fat Fastest

To lose plumpness around and below the waist, you need to exercise for as long a period as possible. Assuming you walk at the same speed, walking 3 miles will burn five times as much fat as walking 1 mile. But the best way to burn fat aerobically is to use interval training. Interval training consists of exercising at high intensity for a short period, then continuing for two or three times as long at a more relaxed

238

pace. Without stopping, you then keep repeating this sequence. Interval training can fill your entire exercise period, or it can last for a shorter period.

A recent study at Quebec's Laval University showed that aerobically fat is burned most rapidly by high-intensity interval training. In the Laval study, two groups exercised on stationary bicycles. The first group exercised four to five times a week at a moderate pace, burning 350 calories per session. The second group exercised only twice a week but pedaled at high intensity for 1 minute, followed by a longer period at a slower, relaxed pace. Although the second group burned only 240 calories per session, they lost nine times as much fat as the first group. The study's authors concluded that with aerobic interval training, muscles continue to burn fat for up to 15 hours after the exercise ends.

Other tests show a similar effect after an intensive strength-training workout, except that metabolism remains elevated for a full 24 hours or longer.

If you live where you can walk up a hill, you can create your own interval training by walking briskly up the hill, then descending at a slower pace. Keep this up for as long as you can comfortably, and you will pump up your metabolism and keep it elevated for many hours.

Since your immune system reflects the state of your physical health and fitness, exercising aerobically and losing weight should restore much of its potency.

Don't Let Ill-Fitting Shoes Stop You from Walking

Many people find walking difficult because they lack the right shoes. Don't even *think* about walking aerobically in anything but modern athletic fitness walking shoes—and well-cushioned ones at that. Nowadays, they needn't cost a fortune. Shoes designed and built specifically for walking are obviously best, but well-cushioned jogging shoes are almost as good. And top-of-the-line shoes sold in discount stores usually have quite adequate cushioning. Shoes with laces are preferable to shoes with Velcro straps.

Make sure the shoe you buy has a wide toe box with sufficient room to curl your toes and for your big toe to lie flat. The shoe should grasp your heel firmly while still leaving sufficient room to insert your forefinger between your heel and the back of the shoe. The shoe should also be sufficiently wide to allow for some expansion in your feet once you begin to walk.

Before shopping for shoes many experienced walkers suggest walking briskly for 30 minutes to allow your feet to swell. Or shop in the late afternoon after your feet have swollen to maximum size, and wear the same socks you will wear when walking. Socks should also fit comfortably with no baggy wrinkles or elastic tops that are too tight. Most walkers prefer polyester blend or wool socks. Just avoid socks made of cotton.

If possible, walk on soft ground, on a walking or running track or a grassy trail. All are easier on your feet than walking on concrete. If your feet hurt, it may be a sign that you need an orthotic, a full or partial support that fits inside your shoe and supports your heel and arch. In most cases over-the-counter heel or arch supports sold in drug or shoe stores will usually relieve any discomfort while walking.

If they don't work, you should consult a podiatrist, a doctor who specializes in foot disorders. A podiatrist can custom-design a pair of orthotics that should correct almost any type of imbalance while walking.

How to Turn on Your Body's Feel-Good Mechanism

Not the least benefit of aerobic exercise is its ability to turn on your brain's feel-good mechanism and to strengthen your immunity. More than 100 clinical studies have confirmed that aerobic exercise is the most powerful antidepressant in existence. That's reassuring news because depression and anxiety rank among the most powerful suppressors of the immune system.

Indeed 35 minutes of brisk aerobic exercise can transform depression into an upbeat mood that lasts all day. Aerobic exercise elevates our mood by stimulating the endorphin effect, one of the principal components of our healing-regeneration system.

Soon after we begin to exercise at a pace sufficiently fast to raise pulse and breathing rates, millions of tiny morphine-like molecules called *endorphins* are released into the brain. Each endorphin then binds on to a pain receptor and either fully or partially blocks out most of the sensation of pain and depression. Once the endorphins are released, it takes only minutes for all feelings of depression, anxiety and hopelessness to be replaced by strongly positive feelings of optimism, hope and cheerfulness.

By also stimulating the release of serotonin into the brain, aerobic exercise also raises the level of alpha brainwave activity, resulting in a calm, relaxed mood that diminishes the effects of stress. Talk to anyone who exercises regularly and you'll find they have a high level of self-esteem and are much happier, more content and fulfilled than sedentary people. All these are factors that strengthen the immune system. Tests have shown that brisk aerobic exercise reduces depression as effectively as psychiatric treatment or most antidepressant medications—all at zero cost and free of side effects.

241

How to Release Your Body's Natural Narcotics

To release your body's natural narcotics, all you need to do is exercise aerobically for 35 minutes at a pace sufficiently brisk to raise both pulse and breathing rates. For most people, this means a level of exertion slightly less than that required to enter the target zone. But it should be sufficiently brisk to cause perspiration to appear on your brow in mild-to-warm weather—except while swimming, of course.

The endorphin effect is identical to "runner's high," only you don't have to run to enjoy it. Any brisk aerobic exercise maintained for 35 minutes should produce the same result. Some people find that as little as 10 minutes of exercise turns on their endorphin effect. But most people require 35 minutes.

Exercising in your target zone, working out aerobically to lose weight or doing interval training will all turn on your endorphin effect, provided you exercise continuously for 35 minutes. And the feeling of well-being lasts all day until you fall asleep. But you can restore it the next day by exercising once again. By exercising first thing in the morning, you can obviously enjoy a runner's high for more hours each day than if you exercise in the afternoon.

The endorphin effect is also a wonderful pain-killer. Many people with arthritis use it instead of taking pain-deadening drugs. Exercising first thing in the morning allows them to enjoy a maximum number of pain-free hours each day. Because of a certain carryover effect, you may find that exercising 5 days a week actually keeps you feeling good for all 7.

Above all, every hour your mood stays elevated also elevates your immuno-competence to a similar degree. For proof, the literature is filled with studies showing that people who exercise regularly have a dramatically lower risk of all

242

types of cancer and of almost every type of infectious disease—exactly what you would expect with a pepped-up immune system.

IMMUNE BOOSTER #9: The Stronger Your Muscles, the Stronger Your Immunity

---

Pumping iron has become the "in" exercise for tens of thousands of men and women of all ages. Why? Because it's the only effective way to burn off stubborn fat. As long as you keep working out with weights—and exercising aerobically and eating lean—your body should continue to look youthful and terrific. Since your immune system mirrors the way you look and feel, the stronger your muscles, the stronger your immunity.

Few people actually lift weights to boost their immunity. They do strength-training workouts because their weight is out of control or because they want to build up their muscles. Strength training is needed because we live in a world of plenty where a myriad machines make it increasingly difficult to exert our muscles.

One American in three is severely overweight because we ride everywhere by car, play golf from a cart, drive a mower to cut the lawn (or hire a youth to do it for us), use a chain saw and a rototiller instead of hand tools, and we rarely ever walk anywhere or move fast enough to raise a sweat or to speed up our pulse. When we accept the sedentary, high-tech, industrial lifestyle and believe that we can live healthfully by substituting machines for physical exertion and fat-laden processed foods for our ancestors' plant-based diet, we're literally buying our immune system a one-way ticket to self-destruction.

243

Age-Associated Muscle Wasting Is America's Most Common Affliction

Most Americans begin to lose muscle by age 25, and by 45, most sedentary men and women have lost a whopping 12 pounds of body muscle. From then on, muscle loss accelerates. Between ages 50 and 80, a sedentary person loses 40 percent of his or her original muscle mass and 50 percent of strength. In both sexes, muscle loss leads to a serious drop in metabolism and an even-more-serious gain in body fat.

As I've already explained in IBs #5 and #6, muscle burns body fat 24 hours a day, even during sleep. The real problem is not so much that we're overweight, but that we've lost the muscle that used to burn fat and keep our bodies youthful. The solution, of course, is to put back into our lives the physical exertion that modern society has taken away. And strength-training is the ideal way to do it.

Yes, strength-training does call for some exertion. You don't have to heft barbells like a body builder and no one expects you to become Mr. or Ms. Universe. But for most people with a BMI of 26 or more, restoring lost muscle through strength-training is key to restoring their health, their looks and their immunity.

Not Only for 97-Pound Weaklings

Strength-training, also known as strength-building, weight-training, isotonics or progressive resistance training, increases the body's lean muscle mass when you work out with free weights or on strength-building machines. Nowadays, it's mostly body builders who work out with free weights (barbells and dumbells).

Most exercisers simply work out on specially designed

244

weight-training machines in a spa or gym. The no-pain, no-gain approach is out. Nowadays, you begin with light weights and increase resistance in comfortable, easy stages. Machines reduce the risk of injury; to change to a heavier or lighter weight you merely insert a pin in a slot. Machines also make it easier to isolate and build up every major muscle group.

For a modest monthly fee you can work out as often as you like at most spas or gyms. The majority have treadmills, stairclimbers, stationary bicycles, free weights, a variety of strength-training machines and classes in stretching and aerobics. Larger ones may have an indoor or outdoor track and a heated pool.

Alternately, if you have a spare room, you can invest in a quality multistation gym machine and work out at home. Or, at considerably less cost, you can purchase a set of free weights with a bench and stand. However, it's usually cheaper and more convenient to sign up at a gym on a monthly basis. Before making any commitment, be sure to check it out during a busy period for possible overcrowding.

Despite the growing number of people working out with weights, relatively few women, or even men, in terms of sheer numbers, work out regularly with strength-training equipment. Yet the benefits are so tremendous that, if you're really serious about restoring your immunity and your health, you can't afford to be trapped in an overweight body that lacks exertion. Work out three times a week, and in 4 to 6 weeks, you should see a distinct improvement in the shape and composition of your body.

Women Need Weight-Training As Much As Men

Working out with weights is no longer exclusively for men. Across the nation, women are learning that loss of lean muscle mass is the reason they're overweight so they're redefining their relationship with weight-training exercise.

Nowadays, one-third of the people using weight-training equipment in any gym or spa are likely to be women of all ages and their bodies are living proof that strength-training works. No need to worry about developing large, bulky muscles. It's almost impossible for women to build muscles like men.

For anyone with a Body Mass Index of 26 or above, this Immune Booster is intended to encourage you to begin a strength-training program. Lack of space prevents describing how to work out with weights or exactly which exercises to do. Most spas and gyms have fitness instructors who will prepare a personal workout schedule and guide you through several initial lessons as you learn to use the equipment. Otherwise, most libraries have a selection of books on working out with weights.

Game Plan for Destroying Fat and Flab

To restore your body composition to normal, physiologists recommend focusing on exercises that strengthen these muscle groups:

abdominals	quadriceps
lower back	shoulders
upper back	triceps
biceps	hamstrings
pectorals	

To get started, you need do only one exercise for each muscle group, making a total of nine. Use a weight that allows you to repeat each exercise half a dozen times. When you can do ten repetitions, increase the weight.

Performing repetitions until you can do no more is called a *set*. At first, do one set of each exercise with a brief rest period in between. As your fitness improves, add a second set, then a third. To give your muscles a chance to grow, schedule your strength-training workout every second day, with an aerobic workout on the days in between.

Should you not have access to a gym or weights, you can always perform a series of calisthenic exercises in your living room or elsewhere. Push-ups, crunch-ups, leg raises, toe touches, sidebends, trunk twists and many others can all be done with zero equipment. Every library has a selection of books on calisthenics. And the results can be almost as beneficial as working out on strength-training machines.

Another alternative is to join a circuit training class. Circuit training combines aerobics and strength-training while it keeps exercisers continually moving at a brisk pace. A circuit typically consists of ten strength-building exercises that alternate between small and large muscle groups. Aerobic exercises are performed in between. The class then repeats the circuit two to four times with a rest period of 1 to 2 minutes between each circuit.

For circuit training you use light weights and fast repetitions. For people with little time, it's an effective compromise between strength-training and aerobics.

Forget about Weight Loss

If your BMI is 26 or above, there's little doubt that the vigor of your immune system could be improved. Your immunocompetence has probably dropped—not because you may be

247

overweight—but because you have a dysfunction in the composition and shape of your body due to loss of lean muscle mass.

By building back your muscles through weight-training, you can improve the shape and composition of your body. As you gradually increase your lean muscle mass, you may not lose much weight at all. That's because the muscle you are gaining weighs much more than an equal volume of the fat you are losing.

As your muscle size increases your basic metabolism will start to rise and you will gradually burn off most of your surplus fat. In the process you'll look and feel better than you have in years. Through a variety of physical and psychological pathways, these improvements will impinge on your immune system and the vigor of your immunity will invariably start to rise.

IMMUNE BOOSTER #10: Pushing Yourself Too Hard Physically Can Suppress Your Immunity

---

Anyone who has been around athletes who compete in marathons or multiday bicycle races will probably note how often these athletes come down with a cold, influenza or an infection after a race. Some athletes I've known always retreat into seclusion for the first 24 hours following a major race in order to avoid picking up an infection. Otherwise, they are almost certain to come down with something.

I've also noted the number of elite athletes who have developed cancer a few years into their athletic careers. I've personally known at least 30 men who believed that a daily 5-mile run would protect them from the health risks of eating a high-fat diet. It didn't. All 30 men had either heart attacks or cancer, and one-third of them died.

Other observers have noticed the same disturbing trend.

Most of us suspected that intense physical exercise for hours at a time suppressed the immune system. But we had no proof. Then a study of the 1987 Los Angeles marathon found that 13 percent of the 2,300 marathoners caught a cold in the weeks immmediately following the run.

Kenneth Cooper, M.D., originator of the aerobics concept, finally identified the immuno-suppression and the excessive free radical production that occurs when you push yourself physically too hard and too long.

While running a marathon, participating in 100-mile bicycle race or doing any similar type of grueling workout, the body consumes 20 times as much oxygen as it does while resting. The result is a huge increase in the production of free radicals.

Part of the havoc that free radicals cause is to oxidize cholesterol plaque in the coronary arteries, narrowing the blood vessels and creating cardiovascular disease. Macrophage cells then move in to mop up oxidized plaque in the arteries of the heart. However, many are actually trapped and become part of the debris blocking the arteries. Then the free radical surplus sweeps into the nucleus of cells, activating cancer cells in the colon, esophagus, lungs, prostate, skin and stomach. At the same time, the excessive fatigue resulting from the intense physical activity suppresses the immune system and keeps it suppressed for as long as 15 days. While the immune system remains suppressed, cold and influenza viruses and other infections are able to escape detection and proliferate; and some cancer cells may also be able to survive and clone into tumors.

At exactly what point in the fatigue process the immune system becomes suppressed is not known. In a superfit man of 30 this could happen after a 26-mile run, or it could happen after a brisk 1-mile walk in an unfit women of 60.

249

This discovery was described by Dr. Cooper in his book *The Antioxidant Revolution* (Bantam, 1994). Dr. Cooper discovered that people who exercised intensely for long periods had higher free radical production, while those who exercised more moderately had the lowest levels and sedentary people produced an in-between level of free radicals.

At the time Dr. Cooper's book was written the best defense against free radicals promoted by intense exercise appeared to be daily supplementation with antioxidant nutrients, specifically vitamins C and E, beta-carotene and selenium. The older the person, the greater the supplementation needed. Since then, beta-carotene supplements have been found ineffective.

Regretably, all research seems to have overlooked the tremendous antioxidant and anticarcinogenic content of fruits and vegetables, whole grains, legumes, nuts and seeds. IB #4 shows how anyone who eats 9 to 15 servings of fruits and vegetables daily, plus 10 servings of whole grains, one to two servings of legumes or tofu and a few nuts and seeds each day should be exceptionally well-protected against free radicals and activation of cancer cells.

For even more complete protection, a number of sports nutritionists have also recommended taking—in addition to an abundance of plant foods—600 IU of vitamin E, 150 mcg of selenium, 1,000 mg of vitamin C for women, and 2,000 mg for men. Heavy exercisers, and those who weigh over 200 pounds, should take 1,200 IU of vitamin E, 200 mcg of selenium, 2,000 mg of vitamin C for women and 3,000 mg for men.

The combination of plant-based foods and nutritional supplements should help protect almost any exerciser from free radical damage and cancer—and very possibly from immunosuppression as well.

In addition I suggest keeping your exercise in the moderate intensity range rather than exercising for long periods at high intensity. In this way, you can reap the many benefits of vigorous exercise without the risks of immuno-suppression.

Among the benefits of vigorous exercise which Dr. Cooper lists are a leaner and healthier body structure; an increase in feelings of well-being and relaxation due to endorphin release, reduced feelings of depression and improved self-image. Each one of these helps revitalize our immuno-competence.

IMMUNE BOOSTER #11: How to Stop Common Infections from Assaulting the Immune System

---

Viruses, bacteria and fungi carry some of the most virulent diseases that plague humanity. Yet many of these diseases can be easily prevented from entering the body. And the preventive methods are among the most simple, elementary things we can do to help ourselves.

Most of us probably know what they are already. But all too often, we become complacent and don't bother to maintain our defenses. That is, until we develop an infectious disease. Then, suddenly, we are alarmed by the inflammation, swelling, fever and pain as our immune system is locked into battle with an invisible invader.

Without medical help, the immune system may not always emerge victorious. Septicemia, pneumonia or influenza can strike almost anywhere at any time. New strains of old infectious diseases believed to have been wiped out are making a comeback. Resistance to antibiotics is growing rapidly as infections like streptococcus sweep through hospitals. Microbial mutants—as the new drug-resistant microbes are

251

called—are a constant threat to infants, the elderly and people whose immune systems are already overloaded by having to battle other ailments.

Diphtheria, thought to be almost extinct, has reemerged in Russia and Eastern Europe, while tuberculosis kills 3 million people a year worldwide compared with only 1 million who die of AIDS. Tourism, air travel and immigration can bring these epidemic diseases into the United States in a matter of days.

A serious infection can overwhelm or overburden the immune system to the point where it becomes so weak that cancer or other opportunist infections can escape detection and flourish. A disease as common as influenza can weaken the immune system and the body so that a heart attack, stroke or pneumonia can develop. Many people who die from these diseases do so only after their immune systems have been weakened by a bout with the flu.

The best way to prevent immunological breakdown is to stop infections before they can enter the body in the first place. The five infection protector techniques described below should safeguard you from at least 50 percent of the risk of infection.

Infection Protector #1: Avoid Introducing
Infectious Organisms into Your Nose or Mouth

It may seem simplistic, but tests have shown that you can prevent 50 percent of the risk of catching a cold or influenza by taking care not to touch your nose or mouth with your fingers or hands. At least half the viruses that cause these diseases are transmitted by human contact. Therefore during the cold and flu season, whenever you shake hands with or contact another person, refrain from touching your nose or mouth until you have washed your hands thoroughly with soap and warm water.

The same strategy can save you from at least half the risk of becoming infected while in microbe-infested hot spots like airplanes, buses, trains, elevators or stuffy, crowded rooms full of sneezing people. Keeping your mouth closed and breathing through your nose helps immensely in keeping air-borne microbes out of your body.

It's probably smart to wipe a telephone mouthpiece in a public place or new surrounding with a piece of clean tissue before using it. It's less likely that you'll catch an infection from a doorknob, banister or toilet seat. Yet you could acquire something as serious as hepatitis or tetanus by handling soil, compost or fecal matter.

It's always best to play it safe by keeping your hands away from your nose and mouth and by washing your hands regularly.

Infection Protector #2: Stay Out of Hospitals If You Can

U.S. hospitals are hotbeds of infectious diseases. Whenever you're a patient in an American hospital, you run a serious risk of picking up a hospital-acquired infection. Being in a hospital is especially threatening for a person with a weak or compromised immune system.

Staphylococcus infections have increased by 10 percent annually in some hospitals. When you include adverse drug reactions, as many as 30 percent of all patients who enter a U.S. hospital leave with a disease or dysfunction they did not have when they entered.

253

Undoubtedly, the best way to avoid becoming a hospital patient is to keep your body and your immune system in top condition so that you will not develop a disease or dysfunction requiring hospitalization. This is a goal you can easily accomplish by adopting the Immune Boosters in this book.

Infection Protector #3: Avoid Taking Antibiotics Unless You Absolutely Have To

Overuse of antibiotics has created an epidemic of new strains of microbes that are resistant to even the latest antibiotics. Just about any antibiotic wipes out billions of friendly bacteria in your lower intestines. These bacteria normally maintain a balance that keeps fungi in check. Once the bacteria are depleted, yeast-like fungus microbes multiply rapidly and invade the skin, nails, mouth, lungs, bronchial tubes and vagina. When fungi infects the mouth, it is known as thrush.

Most fungi are harmless, but in a person with suppressed immunity, about 200 varieties can cause serious conditions in the brain, lungs, intestines and skin. *Candida albicans*, perhaps the most common fungal disease, flourishes in mucous membranes all over the body whenever the immune system is suppressed. It also appears when antibiotics destroy intestinal flora, the bacteria that normally keep candida under control.

Candida normally exists in the intestinal tract of almost everyone. When antibodies kill intestinal flora, candida may appear as thrush or it may cause anal itching. In women, it frequently spreads into the vagina and becomes a recurring vaginal infection or cystitis. Over-the-counter and prescription medications are available for candida. But often candida and other yeast-related infections can be prevented and cured by natural methods.

Here's a popular naturopathic therapy. As soon as possible after you begin taking antibiotics, feed the lower intestines a fresh supply of *Lactobacillus acidophilus*, available in some yogurts or as a dry culture or supplements sold in health food stores. (For more about yogurt and acidophilus, see the subhead "Yogurt to the Rescue" in IB #4.) Simultaneously take a 500 mcg biotin supplement three times daily together with 2 teaspoons of olive oil. Meanwhile, include as many plant-based foods in your diet as you can (see IB #4).

Infection Protector #4: Keep Microbes Out of Cuts and Bites

Cuts, blisters, sores or animal and insect bites are an open invitation for microbes to enter your body. Wash all wounds and bites and clean with peroxide to sterilize. Once any bleeding has stopped, small cuts heal fastest when left open to the air. It's also best not to puncture blisters.

Animal bites and insect stings often carry staphylococcus bacteria that can enter the bloodstream. Almost invariably, an invasion of staph provokes an immune response accompanied by redness, inflammation and swelling. The best natural treatment is to apply hot poultices or moist heat pads for 20 to 30 minutes three times a day. This dilates arteries, allowing more blood and more lymphocytes to enter the area. Although it may take several days before lymphocytes and antibodies destroy the bacteria, the pus from the wound is actually a mix of dead staph and lymphocyte cells.

If this strategy fails, you may have to take an antibiotic.

255

Bites, stings and wounds may require medical treatment for other reasons, especially if you suspect rabies.

Infection Protector #5: Avoid Sexually Transmitted Infections

The United States has the highest rate of sexually transmitted diseases (STDs) of any industrial nation, with AIDS, chlamydia, gonorrhea, hepatitis, herpes and syphilis heading the list. Chlamydia can scar a woman's fallopian tubes, rendering her infertile, or it can cause prostatis in a male. More than 4 million cases are estimated to occur annually.

For both men and women, a latex condom is the best protection against STDs. But even some condoms—specifically those coated with the spermicide Nonoxynol-9—are reported to cause urinary tract infections in women. This spermicide kills harmful pathogens, but it also destroys friendly bacteria that protect the female urinary tract. Women who use spermicide-coated condoms and who suffer from frequent urinary tract infections should consider switching to uncoated condoms.

Having sex with multiple partners or with prostitutes is the principal cause of STDs. Most people are aware that unless the bloodstream is contaminated by a needle or transfusion, AIDS can only be transmitted by direct, moist contact. It also takes considerable exposure to the virus for a person to become HIV-positive. It has been found that women are more easily infected with HIV than men.

While the HIV virus is not caught by casual contact, this is not true for some of the secondary infections that often appear in a person with AIDS as their immune system is destroyed. Herpes, hepatitis and other serious viral, bacterial or fungal diseases are common in people with AIDS. These opportunist infections are easily transmitted through body fluids.

At times, a partner in a completely monogamous relationship can experience an infection and transmit it sexually to the other partner. Though usually mild, these infections—such as the fungus trichimonas—may provoke an immune response with resultant itching and irritation.

But the more serious STDs can cause considerable damage, ranging from infertility to scarring, arthritis or blindness; some can be fatal. Almost all place an enormous burden on the immune system, allowing cancer or other diseases to escape detection and spread through the body.

Having sex with anyone who has had multiple partners or patronized prostitutes is a gigantic risk that none of us can afford to take.

Antibodies Make Bacteria Impotent

Our tears, stomach acidity, intestinal flora, mucous and ciliated surfaces in our nose and throat and the acidity and flushing of urine are all part of the body's defenses against invading armies of microorganisms. But when microbes—particularly bacteria—are able to enter the body, they can multiply hundreds of times within 24 hours, and for a while at least, they can overwhelm the immune system. That is, until B-cells are able to manufacture sufficient antibodies to disable the bacteria.

Antibodies are actually our best defense against virulent bacteria such as streptococcus and staphylococcus. Once antibodies lock on to receptors on the bacteria's surface, the bacteria are disabled and easily finished off by NK cells, killer T-cells and macrophages.

Destroying dangerous interlopers that penetrate the body's

257

defenses keeps the immune system constantly busy. Strep and staph can cause multiple damage to the body. Some may secrete toxins that paralyze nerves; others can cause severe diarrhea or damage to the liver, heart valves or brain. Unfortunately, septicemia, potentially lethal bacteria that live in the bloodstream, are rapidly increasing in hospitals and clinics.

Though we have millions of friendly bacteria in our intestines, scores of other bacteria are crafty foes. They can exchange genes with other bacteria, forming new DNA packages and creating new antigens that may confuse memory cells and antibodies. In this way, bacteria often become resistant to an antibiotic that previously killed them.

You can't afford to let these marauding merchants of death assault your immune system. The five infection protector methods just described are the most effective ways to help keep them out of your body.

IMMUNE BOOSTER #12: Protect Your Immune System from Photo Damage

---

The sun is a giant nuclear reactor that constantly emits ultraviolet radiation able to compromise the immune system and inhibit its ability to fight cancer cells, particularly in the skin. Fifteen percent of the blood is always in capillaries in or close to the skin where solar radiation can create widespread havoc to light-sensitive lymphocytes.

New research into photoimmunology has revealed that exposing the skin to the full rays of the summer sun for as brief a time as 1 hour can suppress the immune system for as long as 15 days.

Nowadays ozone layer depletion allows much larger

amounts of destructive ultraviolet radiation to reach the earth than was true in earlier years. For instance, the ozone layer now allows 7 to 14 percent more ultraviolet light to reach the earth's surface than in the early 1970s.

A golden tan may look healthy, but a healthy tan doesn't exist. Any benefit is purely cosmetic. Despite the risks, 60 percent of Americans under 25 still roast their skin in search of a tan, and the percentage of sunbathers in their 30s and early 40s is nearly as high. Barely half of all sunbathers bother to use sunblock.

By their middle 50s, these same Sun Gods and Goddesses will have skin like that of a person 75 years old—withered, yellow, covered with age spots and as wrinkled as a prune.

Exposing our skin to the solar furnace overhead is responsible for 1 million cases of skin cancer annually, and the number is increasing by 10 percent each year. Most skin cancers show up as disfiguring scaly warts on the face, ears, neck, arms, hands and legs, and the majority occur in people over 40.

The Three Types of Skin Cancer

Basal cell carcinoma is the most common type and generally appears as raised pearly nodules on the face or exposed skin. The nodules may crust over and bleed.

Squamous cell carcinoma appears as raised pink nodes or patches that often bleed in the center.

Both these common skin cancers are easily curable if caught early. A third type, malignant melanoma, is more difficult to treat and can prove fatal.

Malignant melanoma has increased 1,800 percent in the past 60 years, and the rate is doubling with every decade. It now strikes 38,000 Americans annually, about half of whom are under 50. Malignant melanoma is the most common cancer in women aged 25 to 30 and runs second only to breast cancer in women aged 31 to 35. Approximately 7,000 Americans die from it annually.

Ninety percent of melanoma can be cured if caught early, but if it metastasizes, it can quickly become incurable. Melanoma lesions are difficult to cure by drugs or radiation. Currently, the only cure is surgery, and it must be done swiftly to prevent the cancer from spreading. Melanoma hits more women than men, but it spreads faster in men, especially if it appears on the chest, abdomen or back.

Solar radiation is also responsible for actinic keratoses, a thickening of the skin that then becomes covered with scaly red or white patches. While they rarely develop into skin cancer, these lesions are unpleasant and unsightly.

Why the Immune System Fails to Protect Us from Skin Cancer

The immune system can recognize the antigen of most skin cancers but is rarely able to destroy them. That's because the skin itself is a key part of the immune system. It contains special Langerhans cells that initiate the immune response whenever nonself cells or particles appear. But ultraviolet radiation weakens the function of these cells, while it stimulates T8-cells that suppress the immune response.

This process so weakens the immune system that activated cancer cells are able to clone into skin tumor cells while actinic keratoses and similar precancerous lesions are able to form. On the molecular level, virtually all this damage is

260

actually done by free radical chain reactions set off by solar radiation. Wrinkles, age spots, eczema, swollen blood vessels, precancerous lesions and cancer are all the result of free radical damage caused by ultraviolet radiation.

Ultraviolet Rays Kill Millions of T-Cells

All sunlight contains both ultraviolet-A and ultraviolet-B rays.

Ultraviolet-A rays cause wrinkling as well as discoloration and loss of skin elasticity. These rays penetrate deeply into the skin, creating a tan rather than a burn. They are less likely than the B rays to cause skin cancer.

Ultraviolet-B rays cause sunburn and have been linked to skin cancer.

Ultraviolet ray exposure is highest between 10:30 A.M. and 3 P.M. Earlier or later in the day, ultraviolet exposure is only one-fourth as high.

Prolonged exposure to strong sunlight allows ultraviolet radiation to kill millions of T-cells in blood vessels near the skin. As these cells die, the immune system manufactures antibodies specific to their nuclei. In some people these antibodies attack blood vessels in the skin, creating an autoimmune disease such as lupus or an allergic rash such as hives.

The loss of these T-cells can so weaken the immune system that opportunist infections such as cold sores (the virus herpes simplex) appear on the lips. Overexposure to the sun may also be followed by a cold or influenza.

261

Earth's Weakened Ozone Layer Makes
Sunbathing Perilous

Few people under 30 seem to believe it, but sunbathing nowadays is far more dangerous than in the 1950s or 1960s. First, solar radiation damages immune cells while they're gliding through blood vessels in or near the skin. Second, it activates skin cells to become cancerous and form tumors or lesions. Third, it prevents Langerhans cells from initiating an immune response to attack skin cancer cells.

Staying indoors all day to avoid the summer sun isn't the answer. Optics experts have proved that we need at least 30 minutes of exposure to outdoor daylight each day to remain healthy and to elevate our mood. Preferably, we should spend 30 minutes each day exercising aerobically outdoors. People who stay indoors all day, especially under artificial light, frequently become depressed.

The answer, of course, is to avoid direct exposure to the summer sun between 10:30 A.M. and 3 P.M. Stay in the shade if you can, but do get outdoors and exercise during the cooler part of the day. Otherwise, wear protective clothing or apply sunscreen or sunblock. And don't confuse cloud cover with the shade of a roof or tree. Eighty percent of all ultraviolet rays can penetrate clouds. So even on overcast days, your immune system could be harmed.

Protect Your Immune System with Sunblock or
Sunscreen

Either sunblock or sunscreen will protect exposed skin from the sun.

Sunblock reflects the sun's rays, and its active ingredients provide good protection against ultraviolet-B and limited protection against A. The SPF (Sun Protection Factor) on sunblock labels usually applies only to protection against B. Blocks may give slightly better protection than screens and may be less irritating to sensitive skin.

Sunscreens absorb ultraviolet rays before they can penetrate the skin. Most protect primarily against ultraviolet-A, though the SPF on the label applies only to ultraviolet-B. Note that chemical-free sunscreens with SPF numbers contain titanium dioxide which screens out both ultraviolet-A and -B.

SPF is followed by a number from 5 to 30 indicating the burn protection it provides. For this number to be meaningful, you must multiply the time it normally takes to get a burn by the SPF number. Let's say it takes 20 minutes to get a mild burn. When you use a screen or block with an SPF of 15, it will take 20 x 15 = 300 minutes to get the same degree of burn.

An SPF of 15 screens out 94 percent of ultraviolet-B and is adequate for most people. But if you live at high altitude, spend much time outdoors or are fair-skinned, an SPF of 25 or 30 offers better protection.

For maximum protection, choose a broad spectrum screen or block which protects against both ultraviolet-A and -B. For beach or swimming, a waterproof screen or block with an SPF of 30 may be needed. Screens or blocks that contain the compound avobenzone, also called Parsol 1879, offer almost complete protection against both ultraviolet-A and -B.

Apply the screen or block 15 to 30 minutes before exposure. Reapply at regular intervals and use generously. Apply to any area of skin not covered by clothing.

Wear Protective Clothing

You don't have to wear a bikini to expose your immune system to photo damage. Spending a few hours outdoors in a sleeveless shirt, a backless sports outfit or even a thin T-shirt and brief shorts can suppress your immune system by destroying millions of lymphocytes. Even long-sleeved cotton shirts are far from sunproof. Unless tightly woven, most thin cotton shirts have an SPF of only 7, and they allow from one-third to one-half of ultraviolet radiation to reach the skin. Being out in the sun for several hours wearing any of these garments can cause a significant amount of immuno-suppression.

To protect your immune system from solar damage, wear a broad-brimmed hat, plus a long-sleeved shirt and long pants. Choose clothes thick enough to block out the sun; cotton garments should have a tight weave. If you can see through your shirt when you hold it up to the light, it is unlikely to be sunproof. For more complete protection, wear a T-shirt underneath.

At all times, cover your arms, legs, hands and back of your neck. Wear thin gloves if necessary. And use sunblock or screen on any remaining skin that is exposed to the sun. These precautions are essential if you are of Celtic origin or are fair-skinned with blue or gray eyes and light-colored hair. Black- or brown-skinned people have less risk of immuno-suppression but can still develop skin cancer. These precautions can be lifesaving when your immune system is already overloaded, compromised or suppressed by another disease such as leukemia, by an infection or if you are taking certain drugs.

IMMUNE BOOSTER #13: Sleep Your Way to Stronger Immunity

One of the surest ways to boost your immuno-competence is to get enough sleep. That means going to bed sufficiently early each night so that you wake up naturally, without an alarm, in the morning. If you need an alarm to wake up, if you're difficult to rouse, if you don't feel rested and alert on awakening or if you feel groggy and drowsy during the daytime, you are probably sleep-deprived, and your immune system is suffering the consequences.

Depriving yourself of needed sleep is one of the surest ways to suppress the immune system. Some immunologists believe that sleep is actually a function of the immune system. Studies show that T-cell vigor plummets whenever we fail to get all the sleep we need.

For example, a study by Dr. Michael Irwin at the University of California, San Diego, found that healthy men deprived of sleep for a single night experienced a decrease of 29 percent in NK-cell activity the next day. Unless natural sleep requirements are met each night, NK cells may fail to protect the body against cancer and infections.

Despite all this, surveys show there is a genuine epidemic of sleep deprivation among fast-track men and women, millions of whom spend only 4 to 6 hours asleep each weekday night. Then they try to catch up on their sleep on weekends. But that's like dieting on weekends to make up for 5 days of binging during the week.

265

Sleep Deprivation Is Stressful to the
Entire Body-Mind

When a group of 12 healthy male students were kept awake for 48 hours, the activity of their T-cells took a dramatic drop. It took 4 days for the cells to recover their normal vigor.

Animal studies have clearly shown that animals allowed to sleep through an infectious disease recovered much sooner than animals with the same infection that slept fewer hours. Sleep is often the best medicine for an infection like influenza or pneumonia. Observations show that people who are sleep-deficient tend to suffer from more colds and infections than people who sleep 7 to 8 hours or more each night.

Sleep studies show that most adults actually need 8.5 to 9 hours of sleep each night to function optimally. But, in reality, the average adult sleeps only 7.5 hours each night, and people under 40 spend less time than that asleep. The same research has revealed that most Americans are sleeping less than people did 50 or 100 years ago and that the "sleep robbers" are electric light and TV. Today, we assume its OK to sleep only 6.5 hours a night when we really need 8 or 9 hours to keep our immune systems vigorous and strong.

Knowing this, public health experts are worried by several recent surveys, each of which found that most Americans under 40 cheat themselves out of 60 to 90 minutes of needed sleep each night. One Louis Harris poll found· one-third of Americans getting by on 6 hours or less sleep per night, while another survey reported that half of all men and women under 45 were sleep-deficient.

People's Lives Are Overwhelmed by Schedules and Demands

Almost every American under 40, it turns out, is swept up in a self-inflicted epidemic of sleep deprivation. Dual-income couples must juggle jobs, cars, debt, children and chores to even spend 30 minutes of leisure time together each day. Everyone is busy trying to squeeze more and more into less and less time. For many, the only way to get more time during the week is to cut back on sleep on weekday nights and to sleep extra hours on weekend mornings.

As a result, millions of young adults rarely sleep until they wake up naturally and they are never fully rested. In women, a poor complexion with dark circles under the eyes is a dead giveaway of a serious underlying deficiency of sleep.

Damage from sleep deficiency is cumulative and worsens with time. Both men and women lose vigor and vitality and become irritable, forgetful, listless, confused, impatient, morose and even hostile. Lack of sleep leads to poor judgment and a compromised ability to perform calculations. Each of these qualities is a strong immuno-suppressant. When several occur together, they can have a devastating effect on immuno-competence.

How to Tell If You Are Sleep-Deprived

To find out if you are sleep-deprived, lie on a bed in a darkened room around 11 A.M. so that you can see a clock or watch. Hold a set of keys in one hand with your hand just over the edge of the bed. Should you fall asleep, the keys will drop. Note how long you remain awake. If you fall asleep within 5 minutes, this strongly suggests that you are sleep-deprived. If you remain awake, this indicates that you are probably getting sufficient sleep.

Check yourself also on these points:

1. Do you need an alarm to jolt you awake each morning?
2. Do you sleep late on weekend mornings?
3. Do you usually fall asleep within 2 minutes of getting into bed?
4. Do you feel tired and fatigued on weekdays and doze off during the daytime when in cars, at meetings or while watching TV?

Each "yes" answer helps confirm that you are probably sleep-deficient.

How to End Sleep Deprivation

Get up at the same time every morning of the year and never sleep late on weekends. Go to bed sufficiently early so that you wake up naturally each morning without needing an alarm. The simplest solution is to watch TV for 60 to 90 minutes less each day. (For more about breaking TV addiction, see the section entitled "Why We Have No Time for Exercise" in Chapter 6.)

Sleeping the full night through until you wake up naturally soon restores an immune system weakened by sleep deprivation. It also boosts your mood and well-being. A study at the Sleep Disorder Center at Henry Ford Hospital, Detroit, a few years ago found that sleeping an extra hour each night boosted the alertness of young adults by 25 percent.

So what easier way is there to pep up your immunity than to give yourself more downtime each night?

IMMUNE BOOSTER #14: Allergies: What to Do
When the Immune System Errs

The immune system defends us well against microorganisms. But it has difficulty recognizing cancer. And one American in four has an allergy that is entirely due to an immune system malfunction. Whether the allergy is to ragweed or juniper pollen, animal danders, mold spores, dust mite droppings, insect venom, penicillin or food, the allergic response is much the same.

An allergy begins when the immune system mistakes a harmless substance such as ragweed pollen for a microbial invader. Immediately, B-cells and plasma cells begin manufacturing IgE antibodies, each specific to the pollen's antigen. Normally, IgE antibodies are used against parasites. But in an allergic response, they connect the pollen antigen to receptors in mast cells in the nose. The mast cells then release histamine and other toxic substances that produce allergy symptoms.

After this initial response, whenever our IgE antibodies again encounter pollen antigens, the immune response is vigorous and swift. As the antigens bind on to mast cells in the lining of nasal passages and sinuses, histamine and other substances arc rapidly secreted.

Histamine Produces Most Allergy Symptoms

Histamine acts quickly to produce hayfever symptoms. First, it sets off sneezing, congestion and itching in the nose and causes redness and itching in the eyes. In the lungs, it causes wheezing and coughing. It inflames blood vessels. And it may also constrict airway passages, making breathing difficult and labored. Allergy symptoms are most common in the nose, throat, skin and eyes, and they may range from hives or rashes on the skin to hayfever and nasal congestion.

In some people, insect venom or adverse drug reactions can trigger a sudden, whole-body response that can result in death. Called an *anaphylactic reaction*, symptoms occur within seconds or minutes. Histamine is suddenly released all over the body, giving rise to shock that may cause circulatory collapse, suffocation, a sudden drop in blood pressure, a rapid or irregular heartbeat, chest pain, breathing difficulties or a swelling of the tongue and throat. Unless emergency medical treatment is given with epinephrine (adrenalin), death may occur.

Exactly why some people have allergies and others don't remains a mystery. If one parent has an allergy, you have one chance in three of developing it. If both parents have an allergy, your risk is one in two. Despite this, breastfeeding during infancy helps prevent allergies from developing in later life.

Breastfeeding Protects Us from Allergies Later in Life

Breast milk contains IgA antibodies that protect the infant from viral and bacterial infections. These same antibodies also prevent the baby's immune system from overproducing IgE antibodies that can cause an allergy that lasts a lifetime. In any case, breastfeeding prepares a child to have a much stronger and more stable immune system than formula feeding.

Allergies affect 35 million Americans, mostly in their 20s and 30s, and decline with advancing age. Nasal allerges such as hayfever are by far the most common. Although nasal allergies produce symptoms similar to colds, a cold lasts only 7 to 14 days at most, while an allergy can persist for a much longer period.

Colds produce thick yellowish secretions and may cause fever and muscle ache. By comparison, secretions from nasal allergies are thin and watery while the nose becomes stuffy, itchy and sneezy. Postnasal drainage is almost continuous in anyone suffering from hayfever.

The Many Causes of Nasal Allergies

Pollens are not the only cause of nasal allergies. They can be triggered by dusting, sweeping or vacuuming, by sleeping with down pillows or comforters or with pets in the bedroom, by dust from carpets or air-conditioning ducts, by cut grass during spring and fall, by fertilizers or by damp basements. Such an assortment of potential allergens complicates the task of identifying the actual cause of your allergy.

Yet when your allergy occurs can be a tip-off. Allergies that occur only in spring or fall are almost always hayfever and are set off by tree or grass pollens in spring and by ragweed pollen in fall. By comparison, most perennial (year-around) allergies are due to dust, mold or animal danders. Identifying the allergen responsible for your allergy helps because then you can eliminate it from your life.

Doctors treat allergies with antihistamines, decongestants, corticosteroids and desensitization shots. Antihistamines give partial relief. But no medication is really successful. All have adverse side effects and desensitization shots are expensive. The shots work by introducing small amounts of an allergen into the body at regular intervals. Theoretically, this induces

271

production of IgG antibodies which neutralize an antigen before it sets off the IgE response. However, the benefit of shots is controversial and their success rate is limited.

After searching the entire literature, I was unable to find a single natural medicine or supplement with a proven record of preventing allergies.

A NATURAL WAY TO AVOID ALLERGIES

Yet there *is* one all-natural answer and it really works. That is to reduce contact with the cause of your allergy in the first place. Here are some tips.

To Reduce Contact with Pollen

Keep windows closed during the pollen season and use an air-conditioner for ventilation. Change the filters frequently. An alternative is to use an individual room air purifier. Remain indoors during periods of high pollen count; in warm, dry weather that means staying indoors until 10 A.M. That's because pollen counts are highest in the morning and decrease during the day. If you must go outdoors or do yard work, wear a face mask.

To Reduce Contact With Molds

Molds thrive and breed in damp, dark places such as bathrooms, basements and garbage cans. Whenever molds in these places reproduce by releasing spores, they can trigger an allergic reaction.

For starters, store firewood outdoors and remove houseplants from all suspect areas. If possible, also remove carpets and replace them with a floor that can be mopped. Then scrub all mold-prone areas frequently with bleach, or spray with an antimildew spray. And keep the entire house well-ventilated at all times. If you must enter mold-prone areas, or mow the lawn, wear a face mask.

To Reduce Contact with Dust Mite Droppings

Dust mites are visible only through a microscope, but it is their even-more-microscopic droppings that are responsible for many cases of nasal allergy. To control your environment, begin in your bedroom. Avoid all wool and down blankets and bedcovers, and use an electric blanket instead. Enclose the mattress, box springs and pillows in zippered allergen-proof plastic covers. Wash all remaining bedding every two weeks in hot water. And keep the doors of bedroom clothes closets tightly shut.

Finally, dust the bedroom frequently with a damp cloth and vacuum regularly. If you have a bedroom carpet, remove it if possible. Almost always these environmental safeguards are needed only in your bedroom and they should do the trick.

To Reduce Contact with Animal Danders

Whenever an amino acid in the dander and saliva of dogs and especially cats is air-borne and enters the lungs, it can cause an allergic reaction in some people. Most of the problem occurs when cats or dogs are allowed in bedrooms and on beds, especially if they sleep there.

273

To begin, banish the pet from the bedroom for good. Then remove the bedroom carpet and replace it with plastic floor covering, wood or tile. Because cat allergen can linger in carpets and bedding for years, you will probably have to replace your mattress and bedding as well. To save the expense of all these moves, I suggest taking only one step at a time. Some people find that keeping Fluffy out of the bedroom altogether is sufficient. Others find that also changing the bedding works well. Or you may also have to buy a new mattress and replace the carpet. In any case, keep the house well ventilated and mop and dust regularly.

How about Food Allergies?

Molecular biologists have given us a new understanding of food allergies so that nowadays the whole concept is considered controversial or just plain theoretical. Extensive tests have shown that, at most, only 1 to 2 percent of adults have a genuine food allergy.

All too often, what we call food allergies are merely food sensitivities or intolerances and do not involve the immune system. For example, millions of African Americans have an intolerance to lactose in milk. However, it's important to note that cutting out dairy products altogether can deprive a person of calcium that helps strengthen immunity.

Most bona-fide food allergies are to cow's milk and dairy products; legumes, such as soy products, peanuts, dried beans and peas; nuts that grow on trees, especially walnuts; wheat and corn and products made from them; eggs and all egg products; fish and shellfish; and some fruits or vegetables, especially tomatoes. Children tend to have more allergies to these foods but lose them as they mature.

274

Most reactions to food allergies occur within 1 to 2 hours, but some may be delayed for 12 hours or more. A long delay makes it difficult to identify an allergenic food.

If you suspect you have a food allergy, simply eliminate one food group listed above for 10 days and see if your symptoms improve. If not, then eliminate another food group for 10 days, and so on. Known as an *elimination diet*, it is as effective as most cytotoxic, skin or blood tests for allergies and a lot less expensive.

One nutritionist told me that most food allergies could be swiftly ended by switching to a low-fat, plant-based diet (see IB #4); by eating more fish and less meat, eggs and poultry; and by checking any medication you may be taking as a possible source of your allergy.

If none of these suggestions work, and you still have digestive problems, you should see a doctor.

CHAPTER SEVEN

The Psychological Approach: Don't Let Stress Trash Your Immune System

Psychoneuroimmunology is the science that studies the mind's link to the immune system. As researchers in this exciting new field probe the intimate relationship between body and mind, they are confirming that stress suppresses our immune system more than any other single factor. In fact, unresolved emotional stress affects every aspect of the body-mind from the immune system to sexual function, physical performance and self-esteem. Stress attacks our immune system on both the physical and the psychological levels simultaneously.

Stress is actually triggered when a gland in the brain recognizes a situation that it believes to be hostile or threatening. Immediately, it turns on the fight-or-flight response, a hair-trigger reaction that instantly readies the body to meet any threat to its survival.

In a split second, the entire body-mind is adrenalized and plunged into a crisis state. We become hyperalert and every muscle is tensed to either fight or to flee. The stomach secretes a surfeit of acid that irritates the lining and sends people to the refrigerator in search of sweet or fatty foods to tranquilize the pain.

But the core reaction of the fight-or-flight response is the secretion of stress hormones from the adrenal glands. Consisting primarily of adrenalin and cortisol, these hormones are powerful suppressors of the immune system. Within minutes, they suppress the action of T-helper cells that turn on the immune response. And they stimulate the action of T-suppressor cells that inhibit the immune response. They also cut down production of interferon that defends against viruses.

Fear Is the Basic Cause of Stress

Since fear triggers the fight-or-flight response, it almost always arouses fear-based emotions such as anger, anxiety, depression, envy, hostility and resentment. All negative emotions, in fact, are fear-based.

· Immediately when we experience stress, glands in the brain inform our immune cells about the state of our feelings and mood. Within a minute or so, our immune system begins to mirror our mood. Whenever our mood is negative and fear-based, we feel down and depressed, and our immune system mimics the way we feel and heads south.

Meanwhile, the reeling immune system is hit again and

277

again by the stress hormones adrenalin and cortisol. The immune system is now being harassed on both psychological and physical levels simultanously.

Within, say, 15 minutes after we first experience stress, the immune system is so severely suppressed that it may fail to mount a counterattack against an enemy such as a cancer cell or an infectious microbe. The literature is filled with case histories in which people who experience severe stress are hit soon afterward by cancer or by a severe infectious disease like pneumonia.

Imaginary Fear Can Suppress Our Immunity

Anything in our lives that arouses a feeling of fear can trigger stress. We don't have to be attacked by a bull or faced by a masked gunman. An envelope in the mail from the IRS can trigger the fight-or-flight response and create stress just as effectively. From unemployment to retirement, an angry divorce, constantly ringing phones or a traumatic commute on the freeway, our lives are filled with potentially stressful events and situations. Whether a fear is real or imagined, it invariably sets off all or part of the fight-or-flight response.

Caring for a relative with Alzheimer's, for instance, can be extremely stressful. Researchers at Ohio State University, Columbus, proved that caring for someone with Alzheimer's could suppress the immunity of the caregiver. They took a group of 13 women who felt stressed by caring for a relative with Alzheimer's, and they matched them with a control group of 13 women who were neither stressed nor caring for a sick relative. They then took a blood sample by needle biopsy from the forearms of each of the women. Among the caregiver group, the small puncture wounds took 9 days

278

longer to heal than those in the control group. The difference was greatest during the initial wound-closing stage when risk of infection is also greatest.

Blood samples taken from both groups also showed a significantly reduced level of interleukin-1B in the caregivers (interleukin-1B is a chemical messenger that stimulates the healing process). The study authors concluded that stress does, indeed, suppress the immune system, and it does so to the point where the healing of wounds is retarded and the risk of infection is increased

Stress Can Be Chronic

Today, urban life is filled with so many potentially stressful situations that millions of people live in a perpetual crisis state, with at least some of their fight-or-flight mechanisms constantly simmering. These people never truly relax and their life-support systems are in a continual state of emergency.

Chronic low-grade stress, as this condition is known, can be turned on by almost any fear-based belief strong enough to keep at least some of the body's stress mechanisms active. Though a feeling of envy or resentment won't turn on the same intensity of alarm as being attacked by an angry pit bull, any degree of negative feeling—whether angst, depression, guilt or helplessness—can turn on all or some of the fight-or-flight response and can keep it smouldering for weeks or months.

Every hour of every day— even during sleep—chronic low-grade stress can keep a person's muscles rigid and taut while the immune system barely functions. Caring for a relative with Alzheimer's is one example of chronic low-grade stress, but there are dozens of similar stressors.

Millions of Americans live in a state of chronic stress,

279

their jobs threatened by buyouts, mergers and downsizing and their lives filled with devastating social changes. Troubled relationships and divorces take a huge toll on the immune system, while millions are forced to work under brutal competition and pressure as they take up the slack for laid off workers.

Everyone is rushing from place to place, running late and trying to do too many things in too little time. Few people have time to microwave dinner, let alone practice relaxation techniques. Some are completely burned out. A recent Louis-Harris poll found that 33 percent of Americans experience severe stress several days each week, while millions of others are chronically stressed out and exhausted by the pace and pressure of modern life.

There's no denying that it is our high-tech, money-centered, consumer-driven, TV-and-oil-based-car culture that is responsible for the current epidemic of immuno-suppression and unremitting stress. Yet few people seem willing to swap their busy lives for a simpler lifestyle.

Why Stress Is So Distressing

Most of us are familiar with the physical symptoms of stress: the dull ache of muscle tension, cold in the extremities and sweating in the palms and feet and difficulty in breathing, as the torso becomes so tense that the lungs can no longer move freely and breathing becomes shallow and rapid.

The first flush of adrenalin rush may make us feel empowered. But unless we can halt the fight-or-flight response by exercising or by a stress-reduction technique, we begin to feel muscular tension and a dull ache or discomfort all over.

We may experience sore joints and muscles, heart palpitation, racing thoughts, headaches, depression and sweating, leaving us feeling exhausted and burned out. It is these unpleasant and uncomfortable feelings that we call stress.

How the Brain Talks to the Immune System

We've all experienced stress. But we're less familiar with the way in which the brain communicates with the immune system. Both brain and immune system cells contain receptors for three kinds of chemical messengers:

- *Hormones* that are released by the endocrine glands and that travel in the bloodstream.
- *Neurotransmitters* that consist of molecules of acetylcholine, dopamine, norepinephrine or serotonin that carry chemical messages across gaps between nerve cells.
- *Neuropeptides* that consist of amino-acid molecules that convey information about our mood through the nervous system from glands in the brain to our immune cells and to organs such as the spleen, bone marrow and thymus gland. Neuropeptide communication is two-way, allowing immune cells and organs to also send messages to the brain. When transmitted by the brain, neuropeptides carry our feelings to every cell in the immune system, causing it to react in exactly the way that we feel.

Several parts of the brain, including our glands, appear to interpret life events as either threatening or nonthreatening, and at least three of these appear to be linked to a specific part of the immune system. For instance, the hypothalamus

281

gland in the brain appears able to communicate directly with lymphocytes and phagocytes. The pineal gland seems closely linked with T-suppressor cells. And the left side of the brain seems able to communicate with NK cells.

Abnormalities in or damage to these brain areas may inhibit or distort activity of the immune cells to which they seem linked. Or they may cause the immune cells to receive mixed signals, as a result of which they go awry. Then, instead of defending the body as they're supposed to, immune cells attack the body, causing an autoimmune disease such as rheumatoid arthritis. Or a mismatch in chemical messengers may cause immune cells to create an allergy.

NK cells, in particular, are easily subdued by stress. Several studies have shown that students who were poorly prepared for exams experienced significant NK cell suppression during and after the tests. Within a day or two, a significant proportion of the poorly prepared students came down with upper respiratory tract infections. At the same time, students who were well-prepared for the exams experienced little or no immuno-suppression.

The Source of Our Stress Is Right in Our Heads

Stress originates when we must adjust to a change or life event that we perceive as threatening or hostile to our comfort, safety, prestige or well-being. Fine, you may say. But exactly how does the mind decide whether a situation or event is threatening or nonthreatening?

In Chapter 1 under the heading "Don't Let Stress Sabotage Your Immunity," I described how Smith and Jones each responded to the loss of their jobs in a totally different way. Smith perceived the loss as a catastrophe. He saw no hope

282

of finding a new job and soon began to suffer from the physical and psychological symptoms of stress. In contrast Jones perceived his job loss in a positive way and quickly began to train for a new occupation.

Both faced exactly the same potentially stressful life event. Yet it wasn't the unemployment itself that was stressful. It was the negative way in which Smith perceived it that created his stress. The stress occurred inside Smith's head because he perceived the world through a filter of negative and inappropriate beliefs.

This brings up one of the paramount principles of modern psychology. Every feeling or emotion in our mind arises out of the thought that preceded it, in turn, every thought is conditioned by being filtered through the beliefs that we hold in our minds.

Fear and Love: The Basic Emotions

Modern psychology recognizes only two basic emotions: fear and its opposite love. All beliefs, thoughts and feelings can be classified as either fear-based or love-based.

All negative thoughts and feelings such as anger, anxiety, cynicism, depression, envy, guilt, helplessness, hopelessness, hostility, impatience, mistrust and resentment arise when we perceive life through a filter of fear-based beliefs. A typical fear-based belief is "I can never forgive a slight." These fear-based feelings then trigger the fight-or-flight response, and they lead to stress, immuno-suppression and poor health.

All positive thoughts and feelings such as cheerfulness, contentment, faith, friendliness, forgiveness, fulfillment, hope, joy, love, optimism, patience and peace arise when we perceive life through a filter of love-based beliefs. These

283

feelings then set off the relaxation response and lead to a powerful and vigorous immune system, plus optimal health and high-level wellness.

For as long as we perceive life through a filter of love-based beliefs, we experience a minimum of stress. Adrenalin and cortisol fade away, the muscles relax, tension disappears and the extremities feel warm again. The brain drifts into a reverie-like state and the mind becomes clear, calm and free of all negative thoughts and feelings. Respiration slows to a mere six to eight slow, deep, relaxed breaths per minute.

This is the relaxation response and we can turn it on at any time by practicing IB #16: Relaxation Training. In mere minutes, relaxation training transforms the unpleasant fight-or-flight response into its exact opposite, the calming, soothing relaxation response.

Intervene in Your Own Stress Process

Relaxation training is just one of several Immune Booster techniques in this chapter through which you can intervene in the stress process on several different levels. Known as *stress reduction techniques,* these action-steps allow you to gain control over various involuntary functions of the body-mind that most doctors believe can be accessed only by antidepressants and other mood-altering drugs.

But drugs are not necessary. Natural, nondrug stress reduction can be achieved in two ways:

- *Coping techniques,* like relaxation training or abdominal breathing, help you let go of stress by learning to relax the body-mind. Coping is quick, easy and successful, but like a tranquilizer, it works only for a day or so at

284

a time. After that, you must repeat the relaxation procedure all over again.

* *Transformational techniques,* like cognitive therapy, prevent stress from occurring in the first place. By letting go of deep-seated beliefs that aren't working, and by replacing them with positive beliefs that enhance the immune system, transformational techniques can almost completely liberate us from stress.

Supercharge Your Immunity with Your Placebo Effect

By now you have probably realized that our beliefs are key to unlocking our immune power. But one type of belief can empower the immune system more than all others. That belief is the placebo effect.

I described the placebo effect in Chapter 1 under the heading "The Awesome Healing Power of the Placebo Effect." The placebo effect is the immune-boosting mechanism in the mind that arises from a person's belief, expectation and faith in the healing power of a therapy or drug rather than from the therapy or drug itself. A person's belief in the healing power of a drug often produces greater benefit than the chemical action of the drug itself. Call it the power of suggestion, but the immune system is almost totally responsive to the belief, faith and hope we have in any therapy, nutrient or technique we are using.

Hope Is Good Medicine for Your Immune System

Hope plays a tremendous role in stimulating the immune system. Recent research has shown that people with strong

285

hope, and strongly positive attitudes, recover 25 to 50 percent faster from any type of illness, medical treatment or surgery than a patient with a passive, helpless outlook.

Our level of immuno-competence is more closely related to a positive outlook and a hope-filled attitude than to anything else.

Hope enables us to see infections or other ailments as challenges to be overcome rather than something we must learn to live with for the rest of our lives. A cheerful attitude and high hopes of recovery put you in control of your immune system. By contrast, studies show that people with the highest levels of hopelessness and helplessness experience the highest levels of pain and disability during an illness and they recover more slowly.

If you have an infectious disease or cancer, accept that you have it. If medical treatment is indicated, get the best that you can. Then accept that, with few exceptions, no disease is totally incurable. There's really no such thing as false hope.

But hope must be realistic. Don't depend on unproven nostrums or quick fixes of dubious credibility. However, so great is the power of the placebo effect, that some "therapies" work that shouldn't. For instance, a strong belief in the healing power of a sugar pill often results in a 33 percent improvement. Sugar pills are often called *placebos* in medical studies because they cannot possibly provide any chemical benefit. Yet people who believe they are powerful medicines often show an improvement of 33 percent. In all such cases, a patient's improvement is entirely due to the placebo effect.

For years, hucksters have peddled unproven nostrums and remedies they claimed would boost immunity. Some have been promoted by medical doctors and other health professionals. That some worked is entirely due to the placebo effect. Believe in the ability of *anything* to boost your immunity and whether it's packaged pond scum, pulverized fish cartilage or a medical treatment that is outdated and ineffective, your immuno-competence is likely to rise. The extent of the rise will be approximately equal to the benefit you expect to receive.

The Immune Boosters in this chapter—as well as others in this book—each contain a powerful emotional component that can be turned on by your belief, faith and hope in its ability to work. The stronger your belief, the more your placebo effect will strengthen your immunity.

IMMUNE BOOSTER #15: Beat Immunosuppression with Laughter Therapy

---

A good laugh can do more to boost your immunity in less time than anything else. That's because the immune system responds within minutes to any change in mood. And the more upbeat our mood, the more it sets the strings of the immune system zinging.

Recent studies by pathologists Dr. Lee Berk and Dr. Stanley Tan, both of Loma Linda University Medical Center in California, found that laughing boosts the immune system on a broad front. It boosts production of NK-cells that destroy viruses and tumors, and it raises the level of gamma-interferon, a powerful disease-fighting immune system component. It also stimulates increases in T- and B-cell populations and speeds up antibody production.

These data were presented by Drs. Berk and Tan at the sixth annual meeting of the American Association for Therapeutic Humor, a group of physicians, psychotherapists and other health care professionals who use therapeutic humor as part of their treatment. Dr. Tan, an expert on the effect of laughter on the body-mind, believes that laughing blocks the secretion of the stress hormones adrenal and cortisol which are released in response to anger, hostility and rage. Both are powerful immuno-suppressors.

Laughter Reinforces Immunity Faster Than Any Pill

Since stress is the underlying cause of most immuno-suppression, the fact is that you can't laugh and feel happy and be stressed out by immune-weakening hormones at the same time.

Another study by Kathleen Dillon, Ph.D. (reported in the *International Journal of Psychiatry* 15, 1985-86, pp. 13-17) tested the IgA antibody level in the saliva of ten students after viewing first, viewing a humorous film and, second, an emotionally neutral video tape. Viewing the humorous film boosted levels of the antibody which defends us against viral infections. Viewing the tape produced zero results. The author concluded that by making humor a part of our lives, we may experience a permanent enhancement of immuno-competence.

Other later studies have demonstrated that laughter works on a Whole-Person level to produce multiple benefits, including:

- Releasing beta-endorphins that elevate mood and reduce perception of pain (for more details see the heading "How to Turn On Your Body's Feel-Good Mechanism" in IB #8).
- Inhibiting the secretion of the immune-suppressing growth hormone.
- Slowing brainwave frequency and inducing relaxation.

288

- Defusing all negative emotions.
- Relieving muscular tension all over the body, especially in the face, diaphragm and abdomen.
- Releasing hormones that stimulate blood flow and increasing the oxygenation of cells throughout the body.
- Benefiting the endocrine, immune and nervous systems and releasing brain chemicals that make the mind smarter.

Rapid Immune Enhancement

Gelatology, as laughter therapy is known, is one of the few magic bullets that really work. If you could bottle guffaws or compress belly laughs into pills, therapeutic laughter supplements would be an immediate sellout. As it is, the benefits of laughter therapy are free to anyone willing to make the effort, and negative side effects are nil.

Down through the centuries physicians have recognized the therapeutic power of laughter. A biblical proverb tells us: "A merry heart doeth like a medicine and a broken spirit dryeth the bone." But in recent times, the healing power of mirth was first chronicled by the late Norman Cousins, former editor of the *Saturday Review of Literature*, when he laughed himself back to health after developing a life-threatening autoimmune disease.

Soon afterwards, researchers began to scientifically measure the benefits of laughter on the immune system and health. William Fry, M.D., professor of psychiatry at Stanford University Medical School in California, measured the effect of laughter on blood pressure and pulse rate and found that laughter can be as beneficial as exercise and a low-fat diet combined.

Although laughter can be performed on a couch, Professor

Fry discovered that laughing benefits muscles all over the body, improves circulation and heart action and enhances immunity. Many of the benefits listed above were discovered by Dr. Fry.

Put Behavioral Medicine to Work

If you're really committed to building a strong and vigorous immune system, you can't afford to have a downer, even for an hour. Remember that your feel-good mechanism is inside your head. It's not affected by the events and circumstances going on around you.

Behavioral medicine is based on the principle that at any time, we can change the way we feel by changing the way we act. We can turn on the feel-good mechanism inside our brains by changing our physical behavior. Recent studies have shown that wearing a smile, whether real or simulated, can elevate a person's mood. Changing your facial expression by smiling or laughing doesn't merely reflect your mood, *it creates your mood.*

Back in 1984, researcher Dr. Paul Ekman of the University of California, San Francisco found that a mock smile creates the same upbeat feeling as a real smile. Whether your smile or laughter is real or simulated, it sets off physiological actions that increase your heart and breathing rates and your oxygen uptake. It relaxes your muscles and lowers your blood pressure. And it makes you feel good and boosts your immunity.

You can start using behavioral medicine right away. Here are eight natural ways to introduce more laughter, joy and playfulness into your life.

8 STEPS TO BOLSTER YOUR IMMUNITY BY LAUGHING AND FEELING GOOD

Use one or all of the following ways to supercharge your life—and in the process your immunity—with the natural benefits of laughter.

Step 1. Start Off the Day with a Natural High

You can give yourself an exuberant feeling that lasts all day by exercising briskly before breakfast at a pace sufficiently vigorous to release pain-killing endorphins in the brain. Exactly how this aerobic exercise, which could be bicycling, swimming or walking elevates your mood for the rest of the day is described in IB #8 under the heading "How to Turn On Your Body's Feel-Good Mechanism." In reality, you're giving yourself a runner's high but without actually having to run. And tomorrow you can feel terrific all over again by exercising briskly once more before breakfast.

Step 2. Make a Fun and Laughter Source List

Exactly what turns us on so our sides are splitting with laughter is something each of us must discover for ourselves. Slapstick comedy sends some people into paroxysms of laughter, while others are turned on by more subtle sitcoms.

Make a list of all the videos or programs that give you a good hearty laugh. That is your source list of fun and laughter. Whenever you need a laugh, refer to the list and view the video, or play the recording and laugh all over again. That way, you can swiftly have yourself laughing whenever you feel a downer approaching.

291

Step 3. Enjoy Every Moment of Every Day

You'll be much more attuned to laughing and having fun if you turn off all violent and disturbing TV programs and give yourself good messages instead. The good messages you need are such affirmations as "I choose to enjoy every moment of every day regardless of where I am, how I'm feeling, whom I'm with or what I'm doing." Or tell yourself, "I live each day to its fullest measure. I experience the beauty of every moment. I realize all my dreams and goals." Or how about, "Life is just a fun game. To exist is bliss. To be alive is joy. To be here is happiness."

Repeat each affirmation three or four times several times each day while you concentrate on its full meaning. The simple act of realizing the meaning of the phrases can exert a strongly positive effect on your subconscious mind.

If you doubt it, repeat this affirmation as you focus on its meaning: "I forgive everyone, everything and every circumstance unconditionally, totally and right now." Then experience relief as the burden of one or more grudges slides from your shoulders.

For other positive affirmations, see IB #18. Or make up ones of your own. Any one of these may remove an emotional roadblock that is preventing you from enjoying every moment of every day.

Step 4. Say Yes to Life

When you lighten up and laugh at life's problems, they don't seem as big any more. Next time you're stuck in a long line waiting at the bank or supermarket, visualize the clerk with a tortoiseshell on his or her back. Then visualize

292

the woman ahead of you draped in cobwebs and the man behind you growing a long beard. To make it even sillier, imagine the manager serving meals and setting up portable toilets as he apologizes for the long time you must wait. When we say *yes* to life, we can laugh at all the hurdles and inconsistences instead of fuming and feeling angry and upset.

Step 5. Watch Funny Shows

See funny plays and movies and watch slapstick videos and TV comedies that really make you laugh. You need deep belly laughs to boost your immune system and turn on your body's healing-regeneration powers—not just mild amusement. That accounts for the popularity of TV shows like "Candid Camera" or old-time films featuring Buster Keaton, Laurel and Hardy, Harold Lloyd, Our Gang and the Three Stooges. British comedy series like "Mr. Bean," "Waiting for God," "Keeping Up Appearances," "Are You Being Served," the slightly older "Fawltie Towers" series and those featuring the late Benny Hill are also hilarious. So are the modern Dorf videos starring Tim Conway. Undoubtedly, you have your own favorites.

Step 6. The Zen Morning Laugh

While studying Zen, I learned to start off the day with the Zen morning laugh. For 5 minutes, everyone would sit cross-legged on the floor and go through the physical motions of laughing without having anything funny to laugh at. Within 15 seconds, I'd feel so good that everything seemed

293

funny and I just continued laughing and laughing and feeling better all the time.

Try it. Sit down and begin to laugh. If you can't, it's probably because our culture teaches us that it's inappropriate to laugh at nothing. In the West, only crazy people do that. But don't let cultural inhibitions hold you back. A mock laugh creates the same benefits for your immune system as a real laugh.

In fact, Professor William Fry, who has been researching the medical benefits of laughter since 1953, discovered that mock laughter—just pretending to laugh—provides the same health benefits as real laughter.

Several recent studies have found that the diaphragm doesn't know the difference between real and simulated laughter. The act of laughing, which causes the diaphragm to pulsate, doesn't merely reflect our mood. It creates our mood.

When you mimic a facial expression associated either with happiness or with fear and disgust, your facial muscles set off the same body-mind changes that the genuine emotion creates. Smile and your pulse rate drops, your brainwave frequency falls to a more relaxed level and tension flows away from taut muscles all over your body.

By changing our physical behavior through smiling, we can change the way we feel—surely a classic example of behavioral medicine at work. Incidentally, if you're in a situation where laughing out loud is inappropriate, simple visualize yourself laughing (see IB #17).

Step 7. Rediscover Your Inner Child

Carl Simonton, a radiation oncologist who pioneered healing imagery, found that laughter is linked to playfulness and that laughing brings back images of the carefree, uninhibited behavior we enjoyed as children. Actually, it's quite easy to recapture your childlike sense of awe and wonder and your ability to enjoy unexpected things on the spur of the moment. It's much easier to free your inner child when you don't plan everything in advance.

So set aside a totally unplanned and unstructured period each day during which you can create, discover, explore and invent. Throughout this period, drop your mask of adult dignity and stop taking yourself too seriously. Psychologists have discovered that kids laugh 400 times a day versus only 15 times for adults.

For 30 minutes each day, forget you're an adult and play at anything you enjoy as if you were young again. Join a volleyball game, fly a kite, try juggling, ride a bike, roller skate, model with clay, play with children or a dog or do something entirely new and different. Join a class in folk or square dancing, country western or rock 'n' roll. And let your new inner child rejuvenate your immune system.

Step 8. Laugh Up Your Immunity

I've never forgotten the evening I spent in a class that taught us how to laugh away stress. Right off, we each grabbed a hat and stick and acted like vaudeville hoofers as we danced and cavorted to lively polka music. Next, we tossed a ball, tried our hand at juggling, made faces in a mirror and danced, clapped and jumped around. Within minutes, we'd all become kids again. We felt so freed up that we could laugh at ourselves and act and look as silly as we wished.

The instructor told us that it is not until we can laugh at ourselves that we are really in control of our lives. Then she explained that we reach the peak of self-esteem when we can joke about ourselves and find humor in our own mistakes.

That class was the best antidote to stress I've ever encountered. But each of us can create the same effects on our own. All we need is a room to ourselves with a mirror on the wall and some polka music or Sousa marches, and we can duplicate the entire routine without anyone seeing us. When we do that we can laugh ourselves into an immune-boosting mind state at any time we choose.

IMMUNE BOOSTER #16: Melt Away Stress and Tension with Relaxation Training

---

Within minutes, relaxation training can transform the stress and tension of the fight-or-flight response into the calm and comfort of the relaxation response. At least one study has shown that relaxation training increases the number and activity of certain immune system cells.

One 26-week study at the UCLA School of Medicine found that when people with malignant melanoma (the dangerous form of skin cancer) were taught relaxation training, the number and activity of their NK cells showed a significant increase. (Remember that NK cells are able to attack and destroy cancer cells.) Six years later, a follow-up study found lower mortality among participants who had received relaxation training than among the untrained control group. Studies like this have confirmed relaxation training as the core technique of all stress-reduction methods.

Relaxation training also exemplifies the basic concept of behavioral medicine, which is that we can change the way we feel by changing the way we act. In relaxation training, we briefly tense each muscle in the body to burn up the tension caused by stress. Then we mentally scan the entire

296

body for signs of lingering tension. Finally, we use deep, slow breathing to relax the mind. With a little practice, in about 2.5 minutes we can reach a state of deep relaxation and freedom from stress, while mentally we're calm and relaxed.

Mind and Body Are a Single Living Unit

Researchers at the Menninger Clinic in Kansas found that body and mind are so intimately connected that when body muscles are tense, the mind quickly becomes anxious and disturbed and the vigor of our immunity sags. Conversely, when body muscles are relaxed, the mind also becomes calm and relaxed and our mood and immunity are elevated. When the mind is calm and relaxed, body muscles also become calm and relaxed, and again, our mood and immunity are elevated. Almost anyone can learn relaxation training. To begin, you need to know only two things. First, you must be able to recognize muscular tension in your body. Second, you must learn to use abdominal breathing.

The simple methods described below take you, step-by-step, into the deepest levels of relaxation it is possible to reach without drugs. Granted, it takes a few minutes at first to learn each step. But as you do, you will find you can reach deep relaxation in less and less time. A couple of weeks of daily practice should enable you to reach deep and total relaxation in just 2.5 minutes.

First, a word of caution. If you suffer from heart disease, hypertension or osteoporosis—or any form of chronic disease that might be adversely affected by muscle tensing—you should have your doctor's permission before tensing your muscles as described below.

Learning to Identify Muscular Tension

Millions of people with suppressed immunity live in such a perpetual state of muscular tension that they have forgotten what relaxation feels like. As far back as 1986, Joseph Sargent and Patricia Selback, researchers at the Menninger Clinic found that many stressed-out people were unaware of what it felt like to be truly relaxed. Not until they had taken a session of relaxation training were these people able to tell the difference between tension and relaxation.

To use relaxation training, you must know how tension and relaxation each feel. Here's how to do it.

Lie comfortably on your back on a couch, bed or floor rug with a low pillow under your head. Your arms and legs should be straight but relaxed. Place your hands a few inches from your sides and keep your feet a few inches apart.

Step 1. Tense and Relax Your Arms

Raise your left arm about 8 inches off the floor, clench your fist and tense your entire forearm from elbow to fist. Squeeze and tense your muscles and fist as tightly as possible and hold the tension.

Focus your awareness on the dull ache of muscle tension in your left forearm as you continue to hold it tightly tensed. Hold the tension for only 6 seconds. Then release it and lower your arm gently down to the floor. Notice how pleasant and comfortable your arm and hand feel as they experience relaxation.

Without stopping, repeat the same routine with your right arm and fist. As you tense your right arm, compare the feeling with that of your now-relaxed left arm. Keep your right fist and arm tensed for exactly 6 seconds. Then release the tension and gently lower your arm to the floor.

298

Never again should you have difficulty identifying the dull ache of muscle tension and the comfortable feeling of relaxation.

Step 2. Identify Tension in Your Jaw and Face

Now that you can recognize tension, mentally scan your eyes, jaw and face for other areas of tension. Almost everyone can recognize the unpleasant ache of tension at the hinge of your jaw and around your eyes. Millions of Americans experience chronic tension in their forehead, eyes, face and jaw.

You can tell how relaxed you are at any time by asking yourself these questions: Has all the tension gone? Do I feel relaxed and rested? Do I feel content and at peace? Is my mind calm and clear? A *yes* answer to each usually indicates you are in the relaxation response.

Defuse Tension with Abdominal Breathing

Whenever we're stressed or anxious, we take short, rapid, shallow breaths and we inhale as often as 15 to 22 times each minute. The reason is that stress triggers tension in the muscles of the abdomen, chest and neck, preventing the lungs from moving freely. All this is a mechanism of the fight-or-flight response. And its immediate effect is to make us hyperalert while our thoughts race completely out of control.

Centuries ago, yogis discovered that we can quickly defuse stress and tension by breathing in exactly the opposite way. By inhaling through the nose and taking deep, slow belly breaths, the lungs send signals to the brain that turn on the relaxation response.

Abdominal breathing is another name for taking deep,

slow belly breaths. A few minutes of abdominal breathing is all it usually takes to achieve a significant reduction in muscular tension and a noticeable calming of the mind.

In fact, abdominal breathing relaxes and revitalizes the entire body-mind. For best results, I suggest that you try to slow your respiration to four to eight breaths per minute whenever you practice relaxation training.

To begin abdominal breathing sit on an upright chair with your hands in your lap and your legs uncrossed. Or if you prefer, you may sit cross-legged on the floor. Inhale through your nose if you can, and count each second silently to yourself.

Step 1. Place one hand on your abdomen and the other on your upper chest. Then inhale deeply to the count of 4. Fill the bottom of your lungs first, then the middle and finally the upper chest. If you are breathing correctly, you will feel your abdomen expand during the first second of inhalation and the upper chest expand during the fourth second.

Step 2. Hold your breath to the count of 4.

Step 3. Exhale, taking at least 4 seconds and longer if you like. As you exhale, empty your upper chest first and your abdomen last. While exhaling, smile and visualize tension flowing out of your body.

Assuming your full inhale-exhale cycle takes 12 seconds, that works out to only five breaths per minute. This is much slower than the fast, shallow rate at which most of us breathe when we're anxious or stressed.

As you breathe, place your awareness on your breath. Observe your breath as it flows in and out through your nostrils or mouth.

300

Not all of us can slow our respiration to 5 breaths per minute so don't force yourself to breathe in any way that feels unnatural. Simply breathe as slowly and as deeply as you can in a way that feels comfortable. Should you feel nauseous or dizzy, return to normal breathing immediately.

What if you can inhale for only 2 seconds, hold 2 seconds and exhale for 2 seconds? Though that's twice as fast as the rate just described, you are still breathing only 10 times a minute. For many people, that's slow enough to calm the mind and keep you in the relaxation response.

Relaxation Training in Four Easy Stages

Relaxation training is easy to learn when we break it down into four simple stages:

1. Tensing and relaxing each muscle in the body one at a time.
2. Deepening your relaxation.
3. A simple visualization that takes you even deeper into relaxation.
4. Taming stress and tension with biofeedback.

In practice, you simply flow on without interruption from stage 1 to stages 2, 3 and 4. If you are unable to tense your muscle, omit stage 1 and do only stages 2, 3 and 4.

Stage 1. Tensing and Relaxing Each Muscle in the Body One at a Time

By tensing each muscle group in the body as tightly as possible for 6 seconds and then releasing, you burn the

301

stored-up energy that is keeping your muscles tense and contracted.

Before starting, go to the bathroom, empty your bladder and wipe your face and hands with a damp washcloth. Then unplug the phone and go to a quiet room where you will not be disturbed.

Step 1. Lie on your back on a comfortable bed, sofa or floor rug with a low pillow under your head. Keep your arms and legs extended. Your hands should be a few inches from your sides and your feet a few inches apart. Begin to breathe slowly and deeply.

Step 2. Frown as hard as you can and look upwards. Hold 6 seconds and release.

Step 3. Press your tongue against the roof of your mouth, screw up and tense your whole face, close your eyes and tense your eye muscles. Tense all these areas for exactly 6 seconds and release.

Step 4. Press the back of your head down against the pillow and arch your neck and shoulders off the bed or floor. Hold 6 seconds, then release. Then roll your neck loosely from side to side several times.

Step 5. Tense your neck and shoulder muscles as tightly as you can. Hold 6 seconds, then release.

Step 6. Tense your chest muscles as tightly as you can. Hold 6 seconds and release.

Step 7. Raise your left arm about 6 inches off the bed or floor. Keep your arm straight and clench your fist tightly. Next, tense your muscles tightly all the way from your shoulder down through your bicep and forearm to your fist. Hold 6 seconds and release. Gently lower your arm.

Repeat with your right arm.

Step 8. Raise your left foot 6 inches off the bed or floor. Tense your entire leg tightly from buttocks to toes. Curl your toes tightly if you can. Hold 6 seconds and release. Then gently lower your leg.

Repeat with your right leg.

Step 9. Tightly tense both buttocks at the same time. Hold 6 seconds and release.

Step 10. Tightly tense your abdomen and back muscles. Hold 6 seconds and release.

Step 11. Take 6 slow, deep abdominal breaths. During each inhalation, visualize a soft, green healing light flowing in through the soles of your feet, moving up your legs and spreading into every part of your body. During each exhalation, visualize any lingering tension flowing out of your body and leaving through the soles of your feet.

Step 12. With your eyelids open, roll your eyes slowly from side to side several times, then up and down, and relax.

You should now be in a state of deep muscle relaxation. Continue on without pause into stage 2.

Stage 2. Deepening Your Relaxation

Now that you have defused all physical tension, stage 2 uses suggestion and visualization to send you still further into the relaxation response. Repeat the suggested phrases silently to yourself while you create a mental picture of the limb or muscle deeply relaxed.

Don't try to hurry or force anything. Just keep repeating

303

the suggestions and visualizing the images on your inner video screen. Stay laid back and let it happen. In visualization, what you "see" is usually what you get. Should another thought or daydream intrude, slide it aside and return to your imagery.

Step 1. Focus your awareness on the soles of your feet as you silently repeat to yourself, "My feet feel limp and loose and relaxed. Waves of relaxation are flowing into my feet. My feet are warm and deeply relaxed. Relaxation is flowing into my feet and legs. My feet and legs are limp and loose and relaxed. Waves of relaxation are flowing into my thighs. My thighs feel limp and loose and relaxed. My feet, legs and thighs are filled with pleasure, warmth and comfort."

It isn't necessary to repeat the exact words, but give yourself essentially the same message. Place your awareness on the area you are relaxing. Visualize it as loose, limp, warm and relaxed. Or you might visualize your legs and thighs filled with cotton; or you could picture them as limp and relaxed as a piece of tired old rope. Keep on repeating the imagery and suggestions until the limb or muscle feels completely relaxed. At first, you'll find it easier to relax one leg at a time. If you detect tension anywhere, mentally relax it before you continue.

Step 2. Place your awareness on your buttocks and repeat these phrases, "My buttocks feel loose and limp and relaxed. Waves of relaxation are flowing into my buttocks. My buttocks are filled with pleasure, warmth and comfort."

Repeat similar suggestions and visualizations for your abdomen, chest and shoulders and for each arm.

Step 3. Place your awareness on your face and neck as you repeat, "My scalp is limp and relaxed. My forehead feels

304

smooth and relaxed. My eyes are quiet and relaxed. My face is soft and relaxed. My mouth and tongue are limp and relaxed. My jaw is slack. My neck is loose and relaxed. I feel comfort, warmth and pleasure in every part of my neck and face."

The neck and face are very important because tension appears here before it shows up elsewhere in the body. By relaxing the eyes and jaw, you can often induce relaxation in your limbs and muscles. So double-check your eyes and jaw for any hint of lingering tension.

Step 4. Experience the soothing comfort of relaxation around your eyes and "feel" it flowing back into the eyes themselves. "Feel" waves of pleasure, warmth and comfort radiating through your scalp and forehead, down to your ears and into the back of your head and neck and on down into your cheeks, nose, mouth, tongue and jaw.

Your entire body should now feel loose, limp, soft and relaxed. So enjoy the feeling of pleasure, warmth and comfort.

When you are ready, continue on without pause into stage 3.

Stage 3. A Simple Visualization That Takes You Even Deeper into Relaxation

This imagery technique is based on the principle that whenever you relax your mind, your body will also become relaxed.

Step 1. Picture yourself in a beautiful garden full of flowers and shrubs. You are standing at the top of a wide marble stairway. The stairs lead down to a deep, transparent spring.

305

So clear is the water that every detail is visible on the white sandy bottom 50 feet below.

The stairway has 12 steps. In your mind's eye, picture yourself slowly descending the stairs. As you take the first step down, begin to count silently backward from 12. For instance, at the second step say, "eleven." Count on down backward as you descend the remaining steps. At the count of zero, you should be standing beside the spring.

Step 2. Next, toss a shiny new dime into the clear water. Watch the coin glide, flash, turn and dart as it descends slowly through the water. Imagine yourself staying about 2 feet from the dime as it slides, twists and rolls its way down and down, deeper and deeper into the silence of the spring. In about one minute, the dime comes to rest on the white sandy bottom.

You are now in the deepest part of the spring, completely isolated from noise, stress, deadlines, problems and pressures. Here, far from freeways and telephones, all is completely calm, tranquil, still and relaxed.

Now tell yourself, "My mind and body are deeply relaxed. I am completely at ease and in harmony with nature. There is nothing I need or want. I feel only love, peace and joy. I am happy and content, and I am filled with comfort, warmth and pleasure."

Your mind should now be in a relaxed state of reverie. But you should still be wide awake and aware of everything that is going on. If any thoughts of the future or past intrude into your mind, slide them away. Keep your awareness in the here and now and continue to enjoy the present moment.

At this point, you can continue to rest and enjoy your deeply relaxed state. Or you can flow on without pause into stage 4.

Alternately, you could flow on without pause into therapeutic imagery (IB #17) or into cognitive positivism (IB #18). Or you can return to normal consciousness.

To Return to Normal Consciousness: Remain lying down and still. Open your eyes and move them from side to side and up and down. Raise and lower your eyebrows. Open and close your jaw. Then give a wide grin and continue to smile. Raise and lower your head and roll it from side to side. Curl and uncurl your fingers and toes. Then move each muscle in your body one by one.

Sit up slowly and turn from side to side. Then slowly get to your feet. Avoid any sudden movements while returning to normal consciousness and for several minutes afterward. This will help the benefits of deep relaxation last for several hours.

Should you ever have difficulty getting to sleep, relaxation training can help you calm down and fall asleep. Relaxation training can also help you get back to sleep if you wake up during the night.

Stage 4. Taming Stress and Tension with Biofeedback

Biofeedback is the ultimate technique for coping with tension and stress. Biofeedback consists of learning to dilate the arteries in your hands by using verbal suggestions and mental images.

First, use all three stages of relaxation training to become deeply relaxed. Then silently repeat verbal suggestions that your hands are warm and relaxed. At the same time, make mental pictures of your hands as warm and relaxed. The immediate result is that both right and left hemispheres of your brain are saturated with a single message: to warm and relax your hands. Right away, your mental pictures and ver-

307

bal suggestions are unconditionally accepted by the brain. And they are swiftly transformed into physical action.

In a few minutes, the arteries and capillaries in your hands begin to relax and dilate. This allows more blood to flow into your hands and it literally makes your hands heavier and warmer—which is exactly what you visualized and suggested would happen. After a few practice sessions, the effect begins to generalize and arteries all over your body begin to relax and dilate.

The immediate benefit is you let go of tension. Tense people frequently have cold and clammy hands. That's because their fight-or-flight response has constricted the arteries that bring blood to the hands. Blood flow to the hands is then reduced, making them clammy and cold.

Because it creates the opposite effect, biofeedback turns off the fight-or-flight response, replacing it with the relaxation response. In the process, it also warms the hands.

Biofeedback: A Proven Stress-Buster

Biofeedback is widely used by pain and headache clinics because of its proven ability to reduce every kind of stress. Most clinics have a biofeedback lab equipped with state-of-the-art monitoring devices. If you can obtain biofeedback training of this quality at affordable cost, you should certainly get it. Otherwise, you can obtain surprisingly good results from the do-it-yourself method outlined below.

Before starting biofeedback training, check that the room temperature is at least 72°F and that your hands are moderately warm. If your hands feel cold, immerse them in a basin of warm water for 2 minutes to restore circulation, and towel them dry.

Before using biofeedback, you must first use relaxation

training to become deeply relaxed. You can use either the three-stage method just described or the Quick Stress Beater described later in this chapter. In either case, you should be lying on a couch, bed or floor rug thinking of nothing in particular but just enjoying your deep state of relaxation. Then, without pause, flow into the following steps.

Step 1. In your mind, visualize a restful, pleasant scene. For example, you could picture yourself lying in the warm sun on a tropical beach. In your imagination, experience all the sensory feelings, sights, sounds and smells that are part of the scene.

"See" the white sails of several fishing boats on the aquamarine sea. "Picture" flecks of white clouds floating in the wide, blue sky. "Feel" the caressing breeze and "hear" it murmuring through the palm trees. Experience a warm, heavy feeling as relaxation spreads all through your body.

In your imagination, "feel" the texture of the sun-warmed sand beneath your hands and "feel" its warmth flowing into your fingers and palms.

Step 2. Place your awareness on your hands and fingers and silently repeat these phrases:

"Warmth is flowing into my hands."
"My hands and fingers feel heavy and warm."
"My hands feel quite warm."
"My fingers are tingling with warmth."
"My hands and fingers feel warm and relaxed."
"My palms and fingers are glowing with warmth."
"My hands and fingers are heavy and warm."

Keep repeating these, or similar phrases, while you continue to visualize waves of warmth, heaviness and relaxation flowing into your hands.

Step 3. In a very few minutes, the fingers of one or both

309

hands should begin to tingle, a sure indicator of artery dilation. As soon as you detect a tingling in one hand, mentally magnify that feeling. Then, in your imagination, "transfer" that same feeling to your other hand.

As your fingers begin to tingle, tell yourself, "My hands and fingers are tingling with warmth. The tingling in my hands is quite strong. I feel calm, relaxed and warm all over."

If you have any difficulty, focus on warming only one hand, or even one finger of one hand, at a time. If you can warm a single finger, it demonstrates that you have good biofeedback abilities.

Once you can warm both hands, you can go on to include your forearms. Later, you can use the same imagery and suggestion to warm your feet and legs as well.

However far you go into biofeedback, it will take you deeper into the relaxation response than relaxation training alone can. And the deeper your level of relaxation, the lower your stress level and the stronger your immuno-competence.

Affordable High-Tech Aids for Using Biofeedback

One way to check your hand temperature is to touch your hand to your forehead or cheek before beginning your biofeedback session and again at the end when your hand should feel noticeably warmer. However, more accurate feedback devices that measure microscopic changes in the temperature and perspiration levels of your hands are available at affordable cost. These hand-held devices provide immediate feedback to help monitor your progress during relaxation.

One such device is an electronic digital readout thermometer that displays the temperature of a hand or foot in tenths of a degree. Another is a hand-held galvanic skin response (GSR) monitor that measures the amount of perspiration on your skin by producing a tone that drops lower in pitch as your tension level diminishes.

Both these devices provide instant feedback that helps you detect more subtle changes in hand temperature and muscular relaxation than is otherwise possible. Neither device is essential. But either can help you learn to relax and warm your hands in appreciably less time.

Instead of repeating your own silent verbal suggestions, you may listen to a prerecorded audio-cassette tape. Recorded by a professional hypnotist, these tapes take you swiftly into deep relaxation and then into hand warming. Or you may record your own tape. One advantage of a tape is that you cannot easily speed up, or hurry, the relaxation process.

Tapes and skin temperature or GSR monitors are often advertised in pain, headache or biofeedback publications, or possibly on the Internet. Or you can locate them through suppliers such as Selfcare, P.O. Box 182290, Chattanooga, TN 37422-7290 (800-345-1848).

Described below is an alternative method of reaching the relaxation response.

The Quick Stress Beater

Go to the bathroom, empty your bladder, wipe your face and hands with a damp washrag, then unplug the phone and go to a quiet room where you will not be disturbed. Lie on your back on a couch, bed or floor rug with a pillow under your head.

311

Step 1. Close your eyes and mentally watch your breath as it flows in and out through your nostrils (or mouth). Keep breathing smoothly and steadily, but take deeper, belly breaths. As you do, your breathing rate will slow and your entire body-mind will relax. That's because deep, belly breaths defuse the fight-or-flight response and restore the relaxation response.

Step 2. Smile, even if you have to force yourself. Smiling relaxes all facial muscles and induces relaxation throughout the body. Keep smiling throughout this exercise.

Step 3. Visualize yourself hanging from a hook in the top of your head. In your imagination, drop your shoulders and allow you entire spine and body to hang loose, straight and relaxed.

Step 4. Mentally scan your body for any hint of the dull ache of muscle tension. If you locate a tension-filled muscle, physically tense that muscle tightly for 6 seconds and release. Then "watch" your breath carry the tension away.

Step 5. With each inhalation, visualize yourself drawing in a wave of relaxation that fills your entire body. As you exhale, visualize any tension flowing out with your breath.

Step 6. If any person or situation triggered your stress, immediately forgive them. Admit that the stress occurred, but perceive it as nonthreatening. Witness it without reacting emotionally. Tell yourself that by remaining calm and relaxed, you are much better able to solve any problems than if you get emotionally involved and trigger the fight-or-flight response.

By now, you should have reached a very satisfactory level of relaxation, and you can break off here. With a little more

312

time, however, you can continue on to step 7, perhaps the greatest stress beater of all.

Step 7. Half a dozen major studies have identified noise as a major source of stress. In the 1970s, people used to lie in a tub of warm water in an isolation tank, completely cut off from all sensory impressions. Almost everyone found the experience relaxing and restorative.

But the concept of relaxing in silence seems strangely out of place in today's noise filled society. Nowadays, most people can't stand silence and many are terrified by it. People so crave sound that radios and TVs are left on day and night. Even in rural areas it's difficult to escape the distant sound of planes and traffic. Genuine silence is hard to find. Yet only by experiencing complete silence can we really find relief from the stress which is suppressing our immunity.

This step requires you to meditate in silence for 5, 10 or 15 minutes, or as long as you like.

You can remain lying down. Or if you prefer, sit cross-legged on the floor and lean your back against a wall. Or sit in an upright chair with your knees uncrossed and hands on your thighs. However you lie or sit, keep your spine straight. Continue to breathe deeply and smoothly and watch your breath.

Then focus on the silence in the middle of your brain. At this point, you mind will probably churn and chatter with anxieties, doubts and worries. As these thoughts intrude, slide them quietly out of your mind. Ignore other thoughts and focus your awareness on the relaxed silent area in the middle of your brain. Each time your mind slips out of the silence, bring it back.

Within minutes, your mind will slow down, the compulsive chatter and churning will recede, and you'll be plunged into soothing silence. Meditation, a 4,000-year-old yoga technique, can do more to calm and relax the body-mind, and to restore your immunity, than anything modern technology has produced.

Nature's Antidote to Stress and Tension

Behind America's epidemic of stress and anxiety is a way of life that isolates us from contact with nature. Stress is intensified by living indoors, driving cars and watching TV. Being enclosed by walls and windows amplifies stress and anxiety.

Instead, try to spend as little time as possible driving, shopping and being indoors. Get outdoors: walk among trees and on grass, barefooted if you like. Feel the wind and rain on your face. Look at natural scenes and inspiring views. Listen to the wind rustling leaves, the falling rain, a stream or the surf. Watch the clouds by day and the stars by night. Experience the stillness and the subtle changes of color at sunrise and sunset. All are soothing sights and sounds that can help tune out the harsh and stressful realities of our high-tech, industrial society.

Whoever has time to watch a sunrise or sunset these days? Especially in silence or while meditating. *Find such a person, and chances are good that you will have found someone free of stress and anxiety and with a high level of immunocompetence.*

One way or another, you should now be able to reach a deep level of stress-free calm and relaxation. Use it as a springboard to flow without pause into therapeutic imagery, described in IB #17.

314

IMMUNE BOOSTER #17: Therapeutic Imagery: Create Your Own Neuropeptides and Talk to Your Immune System in a Language It Can Understand

Can you visualize?

Make a mental picture of a dog in your mind and hold it for 20 seconds. If you can do this successfully, the answer is *yes, you can visualize.*

Almost all of us can visualize and most of us are very good at it. The ability to make mental images allows us to communicate directly with our immune system. The reason is that our immune system speaks in images and it communicates through feelings.

Start feeling good, and in a minute or so, molecular messengers called *neuropeptides* will convey that feeling to billions of cells in your immune system. At the same time, hormones carry similar information to the immune system and to every cell and organ in your body.

When we feel cheerful and positive, neuropeptides carry this message throughout the immune system, and our whole immune system becomes stronger and more vigorous. When we feel anxious or depressed, these feelings are swiftly relayed to the immune-system which responds by losing vigor and strength.

When we use the language of imagery, visualization provides us with direct access to our immune system. We can create images in our minds that are blueprints, telling our immune system what we want it to do. When we do this we are, in effect, creating our own neuropeptides.

315

Creating a Mental Blueprint for Your Immune System to Follow

For example, visualization is quite effective in mobilizing the immune system to make warts disappear. Dermatologists freeze warts with liquid nitrogen. Even then, they're difficult to remove. But warts are caused by a virus. By regularly creating a mental blueprint in which you visualize your immune cells attacking a wart, you can often make a stubborn wart disappear in 3 to 4 weeks.

Visualization is extraordinarily successful in communicating with NK cells that are capable of destroying a tumor. In one study authored by Dr. Janet Kiecolt-Glaser and associates at Ohio State University (reported in *Psychosomatic Medicine*, 1984, pp. 441–53), results showed that relaxation training and visualization can definitely enhance immunocompetence.

In the study, 23 elderly people were taught to use relaxation and visualization therapy techniques three times a week for one month. A control group of 23 people did nothing. After one month, the test group showed a marked increase in NK-cell activity while the control group showed no increase at all. The test group also recorded a significant decrease in antibodies to the virus herpes simplex (fever blisters), which immunologists consider a clear sign of enhanced immunity.

This study was one of 23 studies which were evaluated in 1993 in an effort to demonstrate that we can voluntarily change the function of our immune system by using relaxation, biofeedback, visualization, self-hypnosis and meditation. In 18 of these studies, tests showed improvements in immune function after these techniques were used.

The studies revealed that most people find it fairly easy

316

to learn to control at least one function of their immune system. One study involved people with rheumatoid arthritis that was believed caused when overactive neutrophil cells attacked the lining of joints in the knee, wrist and elbow. (Neutrophils are a class of immune-system scavenger cells that mop up the debris after a T-cell attack.) To slow down the neutrophil activity, participants visualized their neutrophils as ping-pong balls covered with honey. These sticky neutrophils then adhered to everything they touched and they were inactivated. This prevented them from attacking joint linings and causing rheumatoid arthritis.

The result? Blood tests showed that participants who practiced this imagery were selectively able to increase the stickiness of the real neutrophil cells in their immune systems.

Visualization Has a Long History of Proven Success

Visualization, also called *guided imagery*, has a long history of proven success. It was originally used by sports psychologists to train athletes for world class sports events. Millions of Americans still use visualization programs such as "inner golf," "inner tennis" or "inner swimming." Each is based on making mental pictures of a successful sports technique and then reinforcing these images with silent verbal suggestions.

For example, you can perfect a new swimming stroke just as effectively by visualizing yourself using it as by actually practicing the stroke in a pool. Psychologists have discovered that when you mentally rehearse a sports routine or a dance step in your mind, you activate the same areas of the brain, and you build the same neural pathways, that you would if you actually did it.

Before I drove a rental car through England recently, I

317

used visualization for several evenings to rehearse driving on the left, overtaking on the right and negotiating traffic circles with half a dozen exits. When I finally drove in England, I felt thoroughly familiar with driving on the left, even when making a right turn.

From using imagery to learn new golf and tennis strokes, it was just a step to using visualization to promote health and healing. Early experimenters soon discovered that imagery worked wonders in helping to achieve life goals. You can jump-start your way toward realizing any readily attainable goal by regularly visualizing yourself as having already achieved it.

Want to stay healthy for the next 16 years? Then visualize yourself attending the high school graduation of a grandchild currently aged 2 and you stand an excellent chance of living at least another 16 years. And that means 16 years free of any disease or dysfunction that might prevent your living to attend your grandchild's graduation.

Visualize Only Goals That You Can Attain on Your Own

For you to achieve a visualized goal, that goal must be thoroughly feasible and it must be attainable without the help of another person. For example, if you're 95 years old, it may not be feasible to expect to live another 16 years. And regardless of age, it is not feasible to visualize yourself becoming president of the United States or even a celebrity. But it is feasible to visualize yourself becoming more slender and fit.

When visualization is used to promote health and healing, we call it *therapeutic imagery*. It works in exactly the same

318

way as when you rehearse an athletic routine. You make clear mental pictures of your desired goal. In your mind's eye, you "see" yourself performing an Immune Booster technique. Then you reinforce your imagery with silent but strongly positive verbal phrases and suggestions.

Total Immersion Through Therapeutic Imagery

By communicating in symbol language with the right brain and in verbal language with the left brain, you create an inner dialog that bypasses your conscious mind and saturates the subconscious with your message.

Since the subconscious uncritically accepts all images and suggestions that we make, it communicates our wishes directly to the immune system and also to every nerve, gland, muscle and organ in the body. Powerful inner forces then work subliminally to transform the goals we have visualized into physical reality.

It's important here to emphasize that therapeutic imagery alone is rarely capable of destroying a malignant tumor—it isn't normally feasible. But when used in conjunction with radiation, surgery or chemotherapy, therapeutic imagery has helped speed recovery from cancer, and it can lessen the need for pain-killing drugs.

Therapeutic imagery clearly and definitely *can* boost immuno-competence. That means it can help your immune system overcome many types of infectious diseases. Therapeutic imagery is even more successful when we use it to help change behaviors that are detrimental to the competence of our immunity.

For example, exercise definitely helps invigorate immunity. But if you lack the motivation to take a brisk daily walk,

319

you can empower yourself to begin a walking program by visualizing yourself enjoying a walk each day. Or by visualizing yourself carrying out any of the physical or nutritional Immune Booster techniques in this book, you can swiftly motivate yourself to begin doing them.

HOW TO USE THERAPEUTIC IMAGERY

Call it self-hypnosis, but the brain will automatically carry out whatever instructions we give it while we're relaxed and using mental imagery. The reason is that what we "see" in our minds, and what we "say" to ourselves, is what we get.

In pain clinics, where it is often used to reduce pain, therapeutic imagery is usually referred to as *relaxation visualization*. Visualization works best when we're deeply relaxed. Thus your first step is to become deeply relaxed, exactly as described in IB #16. After practicing IB #16 for a few sessions, you should easily be able to enter a state of deep relaxation in 2.5 minutes or even less.

When you relax the body, you automatically relax the mind and you enter a state of focused awareness. Rather than wander from thought to thought, your mind becomes completely absorbed in your imagery and suggestions. All other thoughts are excluded.

Once relaxed, you simply begin making mental pictures of whatever you wish to achieve while you reinforce these images with silent, verbal suggestions. Sometimes, imagery alone may accomplish your goal and verbal suggestions may not be necessary.

Portray Your Goal As Already Accomplished

However you choose to employ therapeutic imagery, use images and suggestions that portray your goal as already accomplished. To motivate yourself to walk 3 brisk miles each day, visualize yourself as already walking those 3 miles and use suggestions that reinforce this goal.

To recover from an infection, use images and suggestions that show the infection as already healed and gone. Do this, even though you still have the infection. Phrase and visualize everything you wish to happen as though it were already accomplished.

This may strike you as denial. But it isn't. Visualizing yourself free of an infection or disease is not the same as denying you have it. Denial doesn't help. Denial may cause you to postpone seeing a doctor or to fail to take care of yourself. Instead, therapeutic imagery merely supplies your body-mind with a blueprint to recovery.

Make Your Images Vivid and Graphic

You have already practiced a simple form of visualization. It is described under the heading "Biofeedback: A Proven Stress-Buster" in IB #16, which tells how to use imagery and silent, verbal suggestions to induce biofeedback. You have already discovered that, for best results, all images should be as clear and realistic as possible. So choose scenes and symbols that bring alive your positive feelings.

Suppose you have an infection in one leg that prevents you from walking. One of the most powerful visualizations is to picture yourself in perfect health with a trim, athletic build walking briskly along a beach without a single ache or pain in your body. As you "see" yourself walking, use your imagination to "experience" sensory impressions that reinforce the emotional content of your images.

Mentally "experience" how good it feels to be lean, light and flexible and free of the infection in your leg. As you "see" yourself striding along the beach, mentally "feel" the grains of sand under your feet. "Smell" the tang of salt in the air and "hear" the screech of gulls as they wheel overhead.

For example, when I visualize myself working out with weights, I "see" myself lifting a barbell at least 10 pounds heavier than any I have lifted in real life. As I do this, I "hear" the clink of barbells and weights. And when I picture myself swimming faster than I ever have in reality, I "hear" the hiss of water surging past my ear.

If you work out on strength-training machines in a gym, you can still "experience" similar sounds and feelings. Involving all your senses in your imagery brings your mental pictures alive, and in the process it makes your visualization far stronger and more effective.

Picture Your Immune System As Already Supercharged

Your silent, verbal suggestions should be strongly positive. Use the present tense and speak as though your goal were already achieved.

When visualizing your immune system, phrase all suggestions as though your immune system is already supercharged. Telling yourself, "My immune system will be stronger tomorrow" sounds weak compared with, "My immune system is powerful, vigorous, strong and aggressive."

Use only active, positive words. Telling yourself, "My en-

322

tire body is deeply relaxed" is far more effective than saying, "I will never feel tense again."

Avoid suggestions that begin with "I would like to— — —" "I won't— — —" or "I don't— — —." It's far more effective to say, "I am walking 3 brisk miles each day" than "I would like to walk 3 miles each day."

Choose phrases that express feelings and endeavor to experience these feelings as you continue making images. Telling yourself "I am happy and delighted to be walking half an hour each day" allows you to "experience" these strongly positive feelings as you continue to visualize yourself walking each day.

Similarly, telling yourself "Becoming a nonsmoker has made me really proud of myself" empowers this suggestion with strongly positive feelings. You will find this is true, even though you may not yet have quit smoking.

Repeat each phrase at least four times during each imagery session. Say it slowly, silently and clearly. Repeat each suggestion with enthusiasm and anticipation, and avoid being hesitant or reticent.

Ending Your Visualization Session

As you wind up your imagery session, experience gratitude that the goal of your imagery has been achieved. For instance, if you are visualizing your immune system attacking bacteria that are causing an infection in your right elbow, experience gratitude that your inner healing powers have overcome the infection. Do this, even though in reality you are still suffering from the infection.

Always end each imagery session by experiencing deep and genuine thankfulness for having achieved the target of your imagery. Really *feel* grateful and thankful as you repeat such phrases as "I feel pleasure, health, comfort and happiness in my right elbow. I am happy, delighted and thankful that my immune system has subdued the infection."

Finally, congratulate yourself for having taken a completely active step in your own recovery. Tell yourself, "I feel terrific, optimistic, cheerful and filled with energy and hope. As I think, feel, say, believe and visualize, so I become. What I "see" is what I get. Every day in every way I'm getting better and better." These are vital steps in making the visualization process work and for invoking your inner healing-regeneration powers.

Most people can make graphic images that are vivid and clear enough to work well in visualization. But even if your imaging ability is less than perfect, you can still visualize successfully. What really counts is the effort you put into making the images and suggestions and the extent to which you sense and experience their content.

What If You Can't Visualize?

Unfortunately, endless hours of passive, mindless TV watching *can* impair our creativeness and imagination. So if you find visualization difficult, try this. Simply sit down in a quiet place with pen and paper and describe your imagery in writing and sketches.

The very act of writing creates vivid mental pictures and strong images in your mind. So write down your verbal suggestions. And draw simple sketches of yourself walking, eating a healthy green vegetable salad or doing whatever else you wish to visualize.

You can also draw pictures of your immune cells in action. The sketches don't have to be technically accurate. Symbols work just as well. For instance, you can visualize your lymphocytes as vicious sharks, tigers, soldiers or knights on horseback, each hell-bent on destroying cancer cells, viruses or invading bacteria.

Use of symbols in imagery was pioneered by radiation oncologist O. Carl Simonton, M.D. and his psychotherapist wife, Stephanie Matthews-Simonton. Their book *Getting Well Again* (J.P. Tarcher, 1978) remains the definitive work in applying therapeutic imagery to beating cancer by boosting immunity.

The book records a score or more of case histories in which men with medically incurable (or terminal) cancer used therapeutic imagery either to completely recover or to significantly extend their life expectancies. Many of the subjects bolstered their immunity by using imagery routines similar to those described below.

Whichever visualization method you use, most experts recommend two 15-minute imagery sessions each day. For a severe disease or an acute infection, three sessions are recommended.

A Caveat Before You Begin

Almost everyone can safely use the imagery steps described in this section. But if you have any emotional instability, or if you hallucinate or are schizophrenic, psychotic or prone to hysteria, or if you have any other mental or psychological dysfunction, you should obtain your doctor's permission before using any of the techniques in this book.

Since we often "get" what we visualize, never visualize anything that might be detrimental to your eyes, eardrums,

325

heart, brain or any other fragile organ in your body. It's OK to visualize yourself with improved eyesight, but never visualize your eyes removed from your head. And do not picture a knife or nail driven into your eyes, ears, arteries, heart or any other fragile organ. If you have a tumor in a sensitive location, for instance, bolster your immunity with therapeutic imagery, then "see" your immune system destroying the tumor.

FIVE SAMPLE VISUALIZATIONS FOR HELPING YOUR IMMUNITY

Before beginning any of the visualizations below, you should be lying down and deeply relaxed as described in IB #16.

Visualization I: Stimulating Your Immune System to Attack a Cancerous Tumor

If you're taking medical treatment for cancer, this visualization could significantly enhance the success of your treatment. However, it is intended to complement medical treatment, not to replace it. Nonetheless, if medical treatment has failed and you have terminal cancer, it could well increase your survival time. It could also benefit men with prostate cancer when their physician has recommended watchful waiting.

The immune system's response to some cancer cells is poor because our immune cells fail to recognize the cancer cells as foreign. As discussed in Chapter 3, cancer cells are simply our own body cells that have developed a mutation

326

in their genes that causes them to divide and multiply rapidly into a tumor. For example, melanoma skin cancer cells carry an antigen called gp75. But gp75 is very similar to the antigen of normal skin pigment cells. As a result, the immune system may fail to attack and wipe out a melanoma tumor.

Yet all T-cells and macrophages are capable of attacking a tumor if they can be stimulated. That means alerting them to recognize cancer cells as nonself and foreign. The best natural way to do this is to send your immune system instructions through therapeutic imagery. The following imagery steps assume that you have been medically diagnosed with cancer and are under a doctor's care.

Step 1. Place your awareness on the tumor location. Visualize the tumor as a small, weak, sickly looking gray mass. Picture it as something easily overcome, not as some powerful, destructive monster. Then "see" a large macrophage scavenger cell pluck a fragment of antigen from a tumor cell and display it for all other immune cells to see. As it does so, the macrophage turns on a bright flashing red alarm light. Almost immediately a T4-cell recognizes the antigen fragment. The T4-cell produces a bugle and sounds off the immune response. Use your imagination to "hear" this and other bugle calls.

This is a call to all immune cells to hasten through the bloodstream toward the tumor site. Picture hundreds of macrophages and T-cells coming from all over your body to mass at the tumor site. Macrophages gather on one side of the tumor, T-cells on the other. If you like, you can visualize a vast military-style tent camp on each side of the tumor, one housing macrophages, the other housing T-cells. Obviously,

327

cells don't live in tents, but in imagery, familiar symbols can strengthen the power of your visualization.

Step 2. Visualize the T4-cell contacting nearby B-cells. Immediately, the B-cells turn into dozens of huge, transparent plasma cells. Inside each plasma cell you "see" Y-shaped antibodies forming. These antibodies are specific to your tumor cells.

Step 3. Visualize a single killer T-cell. As you verbally count, watch the cells multiply, doubling at each count. Start counting at 2, then 4 and go on to 8, 16, 32, 64, 128, 256, then 500, 5,000, 5 million, 5 billion and 5 trillion. You don't have to visualize the exact number of cells. Just "see" a vast number. You now have a vast army of 5 trillion killer T-cells, all angry, belligerent and spoiling for a piece of the action to help destroy your malignant tumor.

Step 4. After the T4-cell sounds off the "charge" on its bugle, visualize millions of missile-like antibodies emerging from the plasma cells and bombarding the tumor. Swiftly the antibodies cover the tumor. The tumor is now paralyzed and completely disabled.

Silently repeat four times, "The tumor is paralyzed and disabled by antibodies."

Visualize the tumor sagging and helpless.

Then "see" the first wave of killer T-cells and NK cells attack the tumor. Wielding swords, each T-cell hacks the tumor into wafer-thin slices. Next, another wave of angry killer cells attacks the tumor. This wave slashes the tumor into tiny pieces. Finally, picture a third wave going in for the kill and completely annihilating the tumor with deadly toxins.

Silently repeat to yourself four times, "The tumor is dead. The tumor is completely destroyed."

Then visualize the huge army of T-cells cheering wildly.

328

Step 5. Visualize the T4-cell sounding off a "macrophage attack." Picture hundreds of the big white scavenger cells swarming over the tumor debris and mopping it up with vacuum cleaners. In a few seconds, the debris is gone.

Step 6. To end this visualization, silently repeat any or all of the ending phrases listed at the end of this section. Choose whichever phrases seem most appropriate, and slowly repeat each one four times as you mentally "experience" the feelings they convey.

Visualization 2: Boost Your Immunity by Losing Weight

There's a wealth of evidence that being overweight suppresses our immunity. The antidote to being overweight is the "8-Step Weight-Loss Immune-Boosting Program" in IB #5. Visualizing several of the steps you must take to lose weight can be a great help in motivating you to begin a weight-loss program. In fact, you can use similar imagery to motivate yourself to begin any of the Immune Booster action-steps. But if you don't begin soon to carry out these steps in real life, you may begin to feel slightly uncomfortable.

Step 1. Picture yourself working out on a strength-training machine in a gym, preferably one that requires you to do abdominal crunch-ups. "Hear" the clink of the crunch machine and "feel" the exertion in your abdominal muscles each time you do a crunch-up.

At the same time, silently tell yourself "My muscles are stronger and bigger than ever. Each day, working out becomes easier and I enjoy it more. As my muscles grow, they burn more fat and my metabolism rises."

Step 2. Visualize yourself striding briskly along a beach. Use the same imagery described in the beach walking visualization under the heading "Make Your Images Vivid and Graphic" earlier in this section.

Step 3. Picture yourself enjoying a fresh, green salad packed with raw broccoli, shredded carrots, cauliflower, kale, tomatoes and other healthful vegetables. The dressing is completely nonfat. "Experience" the crisp, crunchy texture and the honest flavor of each vegetable as you eat it, and realize that the salad tastes incredibly good.

Meanwhile, tell yourself, "Natural foods taste wonderful. I enjoy food much more when I know it's good for my health and it helps me rebalance my body composition and look terrific."

Step 4. Wind up this visualization by telling yourself, "I am happy and grateful to have reached my ideal Body Mass Index." Then congratulate yourself for having played an active role in your own recovery. And add any of the ending phrases listed at the end of this section, that seem appropriate.

Visualization 3: Strengthen Your Immunity by Picturing a Future Goal

Visualizing yourself achieving a future goal is a subtle but powerful way to enhance your immunity. When you visualize a goal to be achieved 10 years from now, your immune system must keep you disease-free during the 10 years it takes to achieve your goal.

One 60-year-old man, who had already used imagery to perfect his swimming and tennis, began to visualize himself pedaling his bicycle to the summit of Colorado's Mt. Evans once each year until he was 70. At 14,267-feet elevation, Mt. Evans is the highest point in the United States accessible by paved road.

The visualization must have worked because, immediately after Labor Day each year, this intrepid bicyclist has ridden 18 miles up to the summit of Mt. Evans, then coasted back down. He's actually done it 15 years in a row and he's now 75. It's impossible to say with certainty that his imagery motivated his immune system to keep him well all through the years. But there's no doubt that without a strong immune system, he couldn't have done it.

A future goal doesn't have to involve physical fitness or health. It could be to live long enough to celebrate a golden wedding anniversary, or to simply reach a certain age in perfect health. Provided it's a goal you can visualize, your immune system will work subliminally to help keep you free of cancer and infections until you actually achieve your goal.

Visualization 4: Finding Out Exactly What Is Wrong with Your Immune System

If you believe your immune system is suppressed or malfunctioning, and your doctor is unable to help, consider contacting an inner guide for a solution.

To meet your inner guide, simply enter deep relaxation (see IB #16), then visualize a blank white wall that contains a single door. When the door swings open, your inner guide is revealed behind it. The guide may be a person, a religious figure or an animal—a rabbit, wise owl or crow.

Our inner guide is actually a symbol of our own deepest

inner self. Our inner self can access the deepest levels of the body-mind, including our belief system and memory banks.

Once contacted, our inner guide can take us on a mental journey of self-discovery deep into the interior of our subconscious minds and into the vast files of memories stored in our memory banks. A dialog with our inner guide may reveal penetrating insights as to why our immune system may be suppressed and what we can do to restore its vigor.

In one of my earlier books in this series, *18 Natural Ways to Stop Arthritis Now*, I tell about a woman named Betty who suffered with severe rheumatoid arthritis. This is a dysfunction of the immune system in which, instead of defending the body, the immune system's own antibodies and cells attack the lining and cartilage in skeletal joints.

Since medical treatment hadn't helped, Betty consulted a behavioral psychologist. To uncover the cause of her arthritis and how to heal it, the psychologist suggested that Betty contact her inner guide. He also told her that whenever she asked her guide a question, the first thing to enter her mind afterward was the answer.

Betty Meets Her Inner Guide

Betty was instructed to relax and use the imagery just described. When the door in the wall swung open, Betty's inner guide turned out to be a wise old man with a long white beard. When Betty greeted him in silent verbal language, she learned that his name was Porbananda. Betty asked Porbananda what was causing her arthritis and how she might heal it.

Porbananda replied by pointing to a rowboat tied to the bank of a small lake. Betty and Porbananda sat down in the boat and Porbananda rowed out into the lake. Then he stood up and dived overboard.

A minute later, Porbananda's head broke the surface. He reached up out of the water and handed Betty a round white object.

"This is the cause of your rheumatoid arthritis," Porbananda said, "and also the cure."

Then Porbananda slid beneath the water and did not reappear.

When Betty looked at the round, white object, she saw that it was a wall clock. But this clock had no hands and the plain white face bore no numbers.

Betty was puzzled. How could this strange clock explain her rheumatoid arthritis and its cure? Then, suddenly, she understood. Porbananda was telling her that "hurry sickness" was the problem. Betty lived by the clock and she was constantly under pressure and running late.

Her fast-paced lifestyle was creating such excessive stress that it distorted her immune system to the point where it began attacking her own joints.

Betty Acts on Porbananda's Advice

As Betty realized that Porbananda had given her the advice she sought, she experienced tremendous relief. Beginning the next morning, she scheduled a more relaxed workday with less pressure and fewer deadlines, and she set aside a period for exercise each day.

Gradually, over the following weeks, Betty's rheumatoid arthritis began to subside and she experienced a total remission. Using similar imagery, Betty was able to renew contact with Porbananda. And she used her inner guide's advice to achieve even higher levels of healing and wellness.

This story, in which I was personally involved, demonstrates yet another way to contact your immune system. If you prefer, you can meet your inner guide by visualizing a

333

small lawn covered by an opaque white cloud. A puff of wind blows the cloud away, revealing your inner guide on the lawn. By duplicating Betty's imagery, you may also meet your inner guide and discover whether your immune system is malfunctioning and how to restore it.

His Inner Guide Solves Paul's Dilemma

Paul, an older man I know, was told by his urologist that he had localized prostate cancer. He was given the option of either watchful waiting or having radiation treatment. Watchful waiting involves no treatment and allows the patient to continue with a high quality of life unimpaired by the side effects of medical treatment. Since he had heard that radiation therapy could cause chronic damage to the bladder, urethra and rectum, Paul was unable to decide whether watchful waiting or radiation offered the best alternative.

Instead, Paul consulted his inner guide. He was told that the answer would be revealed within 48 hours. At lunch the following day, Paul opened a Chinese fortune cookie. The message inside read, "You can have your cake and eat it, too." Then in the parking lot outside, Paul saw a bumper sticker that announced, "Don't Postpone Joy."

This may all sound very unscientific. But to Paul these messages meant that he could continue to enjoy a high quality of life without having to spend several months taking and recovering from the radiation therapy that he feared. He chose watchful waiting, and after seven years, he has yet to experience any symptom of prostate cancer.

A word of caution: The inner guide visualization is not a substitute for a needed medical diagnosis.

Visualization 5: Blocking Angiogenesis

Here's another visualization that can help your immune system deal with a cancerous tumor. It's based on cutting off the blood supply to the tumor, a phenomenon known as angiogenesis blockage. You'll find more details in Chapter 3 under the heading "Without a Blood Supply, a Tumor Cannot Grow." As the case history below demonstrates, visualizing angiogenesis blockage may really help the immune system slow the growth of prostate cancer in a man whose physician has recommended watchful waiting.

Bill's Story

Bill was 76 when he was diagnosed with localized prostate cancer. Since the tumor appeared to be slow-growing, Bill's urologist recommended watchful waiting rather than treatment with hormone therapy, radiation or surgery. (For a tumor to grow, it must sprout blood vessels, a process known as angiogenesis. One of the goals of cancer research is to learn how to stop the growth of malignant tumors by blocking angiogenesis. Thus far, medical science has been unable to achieve this goal.)

After reading the Simontons' book on imagery for cancer patients, Bill developed a visualization designed to block angiogenesis in his prostate tumor. Twice a day, he visualized a small, weak, sickly gray tumor in his prostate. Blood was fed into the tumor through eight plastic hoses. Each hose was controlled by a valve which could be turned to shut off the blood supply.

In his imagery, Bill rotated each of the valves until it was tightly closed. As each hose ceased to supply blood to the tumor, it drooped and became slack and limp. Bill then cut through each hose with a pair of shears.

335

Each time he rotated a valve he "heard" the metallic grind of the valve wheel turning, and each time he severed a hose, he distinctly "heard" the click of the shears.

Deprived of blood, the tumor swiftly collapsed, and Bill visualized it disintegrating into a heap of black rubble. Hundreds of large white macrophage cells then moved into the prostate and swept up the rubble with their vacuum cleaners.

As this happened, Bill silently repeated, "Angiogenesis is blocked. The tumor is destroyed. My prostate is healthy and clear."

He then pictured the finger of his urologist feeling his prostate and finding no tumor.

Bill kept up the imagery every day for 3 months until his next medical exam. At that time, his urologist reported that his tumor had diminished in size by at least 25 percent.

Ending Phrases

Choose whichever phrases seem most appropriate to the visualization you have just completed. Then slowly repeat each one four times as you mentally "experience" the feelings they convey.

"Where the tumor was I now feel comfort, pleasure, health and happiness."

"I am happy, delighted, grateful and thankful to be free of cancer."

"As I think, feel, say, believe and visualize, so I become."

"What I see is what I get."

"Every day in every way I'm getting better and better."

"I can only succeed; I cannot fail."

"I'm completely healed; I can't be sick. My health is perfect. I'm completely free of any disease or dysfunction."

"I love my cells. My cells are me. We work together for perfect health. We can heal me. And we have."

336

"I choose to enjoy every moment of every day regardless of where I am, whom I'm with, what I'm doing or how I'm feeling."

"I live each day to its fullest measure. I experience the beauty of every moment. I realize all my dreams and goals. To exist is bliss. To be alive is joy. To be here is happiness."

Finally, briefly visualize yourself accomplishing one or two long-term future goals, such as hiking 5 miles on your ninetieth birthday, or attending your granddaughter's high school graduation 16 years from now. A powerful belief that you will achieve these goals is a strong deterrent to dying before they are achieved.

IMMUNE BOOSTER #18: Defuse Depression with Cognitive Positivism

---

Whether mild or severe, depression can literally destroy our immuno-competence. Death of a spouse, for example, can provoke such intense levels of grief and depression that a man who loses his wife is 14 times more likely to die during the following year than a married man. And the cause of his death is likely to be cancer or pneumonia—diseases that flourish when the immune system is reeling.

Researchers believe that negative thoughts and feelings stimulate the release of hormone and neuropeptide messengers that weaken the immune system while positive thoughts and feelings trigger the release of chemical messengers that supercharge our immunity.

One way to measure this phenomenon is to check the saliva for the presence of antibodies that defend us from viral infections like colds. Counting the number of these antibodies gives a reliable indication of the overall level of immuno-competence.

337

Literally thousands of such tests have confirmed that on days when people feel positive about their lives and themselves, their immune function is much stronger than on days when they feel melancholy or depressed. When blood samples are taken in addition, they invariably show a higher ratio of T-helper cells to T-suppressor cells in people who are optimistic. (T-helper cells turn on the immune response while T-suppressor cells turn it off.)

How Worn-out Beliefs Suppress Our Immunity

Mild-to-moderate depression—the type we're concerned with here—is usually due to psychological causes such as holding inappropriate beliefs. Since we perceive the world through a filter of our beliefs, our thoughts and emotions are strongly colored by those beliefs. Holding negative beliefs provokes negative thoughts that trigger negative emotions such as anger, anxiety, envy, fear, guilt, helplessness, hopelessness, hostility, impatience, mistrust, resentment and sadness. Emotions like these cause us to:

Feel irritable much of the day.

Lose interest or pleasure in most activities.

Experience a change in weight or appetite.

Sleep more or fewer hours than normal.

Experience unusual levels of agitation, fatigue or restlessness and slowing of motor skills.

Feel despairing, helpless, hopeless and worthless.

338

Experience an impairment in concentration and in cognitive abilities.

Think about suicide and death.

These, incidentally, are the symptoms of depression and they can sap all a person's hope, pleasure and vitality. They may also be symptoms of at least 15 different medical conditions, or they may be due to the side effects of common prescription drugs. To rule out these possibilities, you should always consult a physician before concluding that you have depression

Moderate-to-severe depression, also known as *clinical depression*, is usually due to a preexisting imbalance of chemicals in the brain. It requires medical treatment, usually in the form of a powerful antidepressant such as Prozac. Common side effects of antidepressant medications include anxiety, appetite loss, breathing difficulty, dizziness, drowsiness, headaches, insomnia, loss of coordination, problems in urinating, rapid pulse, rash, restlessness and sexual problems.

Both mild and severe depression are twice as common in women as in men. The main difference is that mild-to-moderate psychologically induced depression can usually be reversed by simple do-it-yourself mind techniques like those described below.

First, however, here are three simple remedies that may often chase the blues away in 30 to 60 minutes.

339

THREE SIMPLE REMEDIES FOR CHASING AWAY THE BLUES

Mood Booster I

Simply eat two ripe bananas, especially ones that are speckled with brown dots, indicating they are perfectly ripe. Bananas like these release serotonin and norepinephrine that work together to raise your spirits. They may be even more effective when the bananas are spread on a slice of 100 percent whole grain bread. (Be sure not to eat bananas that are bruised or rotten.)

Mood Booster 2

Exercising briskly for 35 minutes is the swiftest and surest natural mood booster. More than 100 studies have confirmed that brisk aerobic exercise such as walking releases clouds of feel-good neurotransmitters in the brain called endorphins. These morphine-like molecules block pain receptors, making it difficult to experience anxiety, depression, malaise or restlessness. They are also powerful boosters of self-esteem. People who exercise every day are always much happier and are invariably optimists.

Since the benefits of endorphins last all day until you fall asleep, the earlier in the day you exercise, the longer you can enjoy feeling good. The next day, you can recapture all your positive feelings by exercising once again.

Mood Booster 3

Sit down and begin abdominal breathing as described in IB #16 under the heading "Defuse Tension with Abdominal Breathing." With each inhalation, picture calm, happy feelings flowing into your body while fear and other negative emotions leave the body with each exhalation. If you're mad at someone, imagine forgiveness entering with each inhalation and resentment flowing out with each exhalation For easier visualization, imagine forgiveness as a blue cloud and resentment as a red cloud. Then simply watch your breath for a few minutes as it flows in and out.

You can also prevent downer moods by ensuring that your vitamin-B intake is complete. Besides bananas, ripe avocadoes and legumes contain nutrients that help dispel depression. Vitamin-B deficiency occurs in 75 percent of people with depression compared with only 30 percent of healthy people.

You can prevent a B-vitamin deficiency by taking a broad-spectrum B-vitamin supplement each day. Some nutritionists have also advised avoiding polyunsaturated cooking oils like soy and corn oil. Both are rich in omega-6 fatty acids, known to deepen depression in many people. In contrast, fatty fish like Atlantic or sockeye salmon, bluefish, halibut, herring and mackerel are rich in omega-3 fatty acids, which studies have shown help prevent depression.

Pessimism Is Bad News for the Immune System

Basically, we're all either optimists or pessimists. Pessimism is widespread among all ages in the United States. A

341

pessimistic person typically holds negative beliefs such as that the future will be worse than now, with greater crime, drugs, environmental destruction and joblessness. With such an outlook, life seems meaningless, unfair, unfulfilling and unsatisfying. Almost always, a person who holds such beliefs suffers from depression and experiences a steep decline in immuno-competence, with adverse effects on health and well-being.

By contrast, an optimist expects everything to succeed and turn out well. If a setback does occur, it is viewed as merely a minor, temporary mistake from which lessons can be learned. Optimists typically believe that good things will happen to them today and in the future. They are confident of success. And they take complete responsibility for their health and for whatever happens to them. Obviously, optimists enjoy a high level of immuno-competence and they experience a healthy and disease-free lifestyle.

The message of this Immune Booster is that if your depression is psychologically caused, you can easily transform yourself from a pessimist to an optimist by restructuring your beliefs. The good news is that you're not stuck with a pessimistic personality. If you're not satisfied with your personality configuration, you can easily change it through a system of belief reprogramming known as *cognitive positivism*.

Build a New Personality with Cognitive Positivism

You can learn cognitive positivism in two easy stages:

Stage 1. *Cognitive training,* as it's also called, helps you identify distortions in your thinking process that cause depression. Then you learn to reframe your thoughts more appropriately so that the outcome is positive.

342

Stage 2. *Belief restructuring*, as this stage is also known, shows how to overlay old, worn-out beliefs that cause depression with new, positive beliefs that trigger optimism and wellness.

Merely knowing that you can overcome psychologically induced depression with these action-steps can be a powerful booster to your placebo and enabling effects and to your immuno-competence.

And while we're focused on beating depression, these very same techniques can transform stress into nonstress. So cognitive positivism gives you a really big bang for your buck.

Here's how to get started.

STAGE 1: COGNITIVE TRAINING

Originally discovered by David Burns, M.D., associate professor of psychiatry at the University of Pennsylvania School of Medicine, cognitive training is now the most widely used natural therapy for treating depression. Experience shows that it relieves mild-to-moderate depression in approximately 70 percent of people whose depression is psychologically induced. Typically, it takes about a month of regular daily use for positive results to appear.

You begin cognitive training by identifying the 10 most common ways in which distorted thinking causes you to view life negatively. These inappropriate ways of thinking are each described below so that you can easily recognize them in your own thinking process. As we allow these negative assumptions to color our world view, they trigger thoughts of failure, helplessness and every other aspect of depression.

You then learn how to replace and reframe these distorted assumptions in a more accurate and appropriate way. Tests have shown that for psychologically induced depression, cognitive training is as effective as most drug therapy.

The Ten Most Common Variations of Distorted Thinking

1. Making a mountain out of a molehill.
2. Holding on to all-or-nothing thinking in which you see yourself as a total failure if your performance fails to measure up in just one area, even though you may have succeeded everywhere else.
3. Exaggerating a minor drawback, while ignoring an overwhelming number of advantages.
4. Prefacing your thoughts with "I must," "I should," "I ought to" or "I should not." This approach is an almost guaranteed way to distort your thinking processes.
5. Ignoring positive factors while you zero in on negative aspects.
6. Jumping to a negative conclusion even when there are no facts to support it.
7. Seeing yourself as responsible for something when you are not.
8. Viewing a single negative aspect as an endlessly repeated pattern of defeat.
9. Allowing yourself to be run by the way you feel rather than by logical thinking.
10. Perceiving yourself and others negatively. For example, you may regard yourself as a "loser." Or if someone else's behavior rubs you the wrong way, you might label him or her as "dysfunctional"—without any real justification.

Any one or a combination of these irrational ways of thinking can trigger stress, or lead a person into depression or anxiety.

344

Cognitive training begins by having you look inward for the source of your depression. What you feel stressed or depressed about is unimportant. What counts is how your mind is *processing* the information.

Robert Beats Depression Caused by Distorted Thinking

For instance, Robert bought a used car that seemed plagued by problems. First, the radio and tape player went dead. Then the windshield wipers quit in the middle of a heavy rainstorm on a busy freeway. Finally, the car refused to start. Other than these things, the car seemed in unusually good condition, with plenty of pickup and power.

But Robert didn't see it that way.

"In three days I've had three different breakdowns," he complained. "This car's a real lemon. I've thrown away my money."

However, when a mechanic checked the car he found only one problem, a faulty ignition switch. This switch had been responsible for all three failures that Robert experienced.

But even after the switch was replaced, Robert continued to regard the car as worthless. He felt so depressed and unhappy that he consulted a psychologist. Right away, the psychologist told Robert to stop thinking about the car.

"It isn't the car that's making you depressed," the therapist said. "It's the way your mind is distorting the facts."

As the therapist explained, Robert was experiencing not merely one type of distorted thinking but several. For example, he was making a mountain out of a molehill, allowing himself to be run by the way he felt, jumping to a conclusion without supporting facts, ignoring positive factors while

345

focusing on negative points, and exaggerating a minor drawback while ignoring an overwhelming number of advantages.

"Your thinking is so distorted that it has blown up a single, small flaw in your car into a huge generalization that the entire car is worthless," the therapist went on. "Today it's your car. Tomorrow it could be your finances, your job or your relationships. Your mind is negatively programmed so that you continually see the world in a distorted way. Instead of a safe, nonthreatening world out there, you see everything as negative and threatening."

Once Robert learned to recognize when his thinking was distorted, it only took a few weeks for all traces of stress and depression to disappear.

How Brenda Reprogrammed Her All-or-Nothing Thinking Pattern

Whenever Brenda experienced a small setback, she immediately reacted by thinking that nothing she ever did was right. A friend who was familiar with cognitive training explained to Brenda that her problem was a clear-cut example of all-or-nothing thinking. Or, put another way, she exaggerated a minor drawback while ignoring an overwhelming number of advantages.

Her friend told Brenda to make a list of everything she had going for her: her achievements, talents, experience and any other successes in hobbies, investing, relationships or sports. Whenever she saw herself as a failure, Brenda was to read her list of successes and then to mentally magnify these feelings of success into her entire life.

After a few tries, Brenda found that this simple exercise swiftly canceled out any tendency to generalize a single negative aspect. Never again did she tell herself, "I can't succeed at anything."

A Single Mistake Doesn't Mean Total Failure

Jack frequently felt depressed about the way he handled situations that occurred in his life. After reading a book on cognitive training, he learned that whenever this occurred, he was to:

1. Write down three responses to the situation that might have been better.
2. Write down three responses that might have been worse.
3. Think of a person whose coping skills he admired. Then consider how he or she might have handled the situation and describe it in writing.

This simple exercise quickly straightened out Jack's distorted thinking and demonstrated that a single mistake didn't mean he was a total failure. Above all, the exercise boosted his confidence to where he was able to handle future situations without feeling stressed or depressed.

Catastrophic Thinking Can Suppress Your Immunity

We haven't mentioned immunity lately but stress and depression are synonymous with immuno-suppression. And catastrophic thinking can have a devastating effect on the immune system. Catastrophic thinking is when we react to something by saying, "This is the worst thing that ever happened to me."

347

But are you certain that it's really a catastrophe? Or are you making a mountain out of a molehill? It's easy to magnify a relatively insignificant problem into a crisis.

So check your facts again. Chances are that the risk of a real catastrophe is small. Ninety percent of what we worry about never really happens. As one woman aptly put it, "Don't sweat the small stuff. It's all small stuff."

STAGE 2: BELIEF RESTRUCTURING

Our beliefs mould our personality and they make us who we are. But the wonderful thing is that if we aren't satisfied with our personality configuration, we can easily change it. If we have a negative personality, prone to stress and depression, we can easily transform it into a positive, stress-free personality by restructuring our beliefs.

How? By overlaying the worn-out, negative beliefs that we hold in our minds with new, positive beliefs that can boost our immunity and upgrade our health.

Since most of us have no way of measuring our immunocompetence, it's difficult to show how we can send our immunity soaring by adopting new, optimistic beliefs. Instead, I'd like to quote a case history from an earlier book in this series, *18 Natural Ways to Stop Arthritis Now.*

Rheumatoid arthritis develops when stress and depression distort the immune system, causing it to attack the lining and cartilage of the body's own joints. One of the major causes of stress and depression (and, therefore, of rheumatoid arthritis) is the belief that we should never forgive a slight.

A Single Positive Belief Gives Karen Control
of Her Immunity

In our violent and competitive society, millions of people have grown up believing that to forgive someone is wimpish. Karen had typically grown up with the belief that she should never forgive an injustice. Karen felt badly cheated when, instead of promoting her to the job for which she was next in line, her boss gave the job to his niece, a young college graduate with no work experience.

Whenever Karen thought about how unjustly she had been treated, she would immediately feel tense and uncomfortable. But she saw no reason to forgive her boss, and she continued to feel resentful week after week.

One morning when Karen woke up, her wrists seemed on fire. Her doctor diagnosed it as rheumatoid arthritis and prescribed a series of pain-killing drugs. Despite this, the pain spread into Karen's shoulders and her arthritis slowly worsened.

While waiting in her doctor's office one day, Karen read an article in a health magazine about behavioral medicine. The author explained how negative emotions like fear and resentment could suppress or distort the immune system and provoke cancer or rheumatoid arthritis. Though far from convinced, Karen phoned the 800 number quoted in the article and located a behavioral psychologist in her city.

The Wonder Working Power of Behavioral
Psychology

A week later, Karen was seated in the psychologist's office describing her arthritis symptoms. The psychologist didn't

349

seem too interested in Karen's physical symptoms. Instead, she asked Karen whom she was mad at.

"My boss, of course," Karen blurted out. "I've been treated most unjustly. I've worked for his company for almost eight years. I was next in line for promotion to department head. But instead of giving me the job, my boss gave it to his niece who has no experience and is fresh out of college. It makes me furious just to think about it. I'll never forgive him. Somebody's going to pay for this."

The psychologist looked straight at Karen. "Somebody already *is* paying for it," she told Karen. *"You are."*

Karen had difficulty accepting that it was her resentment and unforgiveness that distorted her immune system and triggered the arthritis.

"Forgive your boss," the psychologist said. "I mean *really* forgive him. What have you to lose but your arthritis and all the inappropriate beliefs you've been carrying around in your mind for years? Whether an act is just or unjust depends on how you look at it. Condemning your boss didn't hurt him. You are the one who's suffered. It's your negative beliefs, and the destructive emotions they produced, that are causing your arthritis."

Karen felt angry at this explanation. But something deep inside told her that the psychologist was right.

"I know these beliefs are destroying me," Karen admitted. "Can you help me forgive my boss and get rid of my arthritis?"

During the next hour, Karen learned the basics of relaxation and therapeutic imagery. The psychologist then taught her a therapeutic imagery technique specifically designed for restructuring beliefs.

Assuming you have already learned how to use deep relaxation (IB #16) and therapeutic imagery (IB #17), you can

350

begin using the therapeutic imagery technique right away. The description below assumes that you do not know exactly which negative belief you should drop and which positive belief you should adopt in its place. However, the technique works just as well with beliefs you are already aware of.

A Powerful Zen Visualization for Restructuring Beliefs

To replace a negative belief in your mind with a positive belief, imagine yourself in a Zen temple in Japan. Picture yourself sitting cross-legged on the tatami-mat floor. Immediately in front of you, a flame is burning on a low brass pedestal. Mentally, you "smell" the perfume of burning incense and you "hear" the temple bells and the chanting of monks in the distance.

Step 1. First, you destroy the negative belief that is causing your stress and depression. On the floor to your left is a rolled-up scroll; pick it up and unroll it. Written inside, in English, is the negative belief that is suppressing your immunity.

Typically, it might read: "I'll never forgive my sister for what she did to me."

Picture yourself holding the scroll over the flame and watch it burn. "Smell" the paper burning.

A monk with a shaved head and wearing a brown robe comes forward. In his hands is a brass bowl. You empty the ashes into the bowl and the monk withdraws.

Step 2. Next, you install a new, positive belief in your mind. To your right, see another scroll lying on the floor. Pick it

351

up and unroll it. The scroll is blank. Using a thick marker pen, write the new belief to be installed in your mind. The new belief is the first thing that enters your head. You might write, for example: "I forgive my sister now, always, totally and unconditionally. I also forgive myself for having judged her in the first place."

What your sister did or how unjust it seemed are irrelevant. You don't have to see or contact her. Simply forgive her. The alternative is to continue to experience the depression that is suppressing your immunity.

Read your new belief slowly three times as you absorb it and experience it.

Once more the monk comes forward and takes the scroll. "The new belief is etched in your memory," he tells you as he leaves. "It will remain there forever."

Zen Imagery Helps Karen Restore Balance to Her Immunity

Using the Zen technique, Karen was able to completely forgive her boss after just two sessions. As she let go of her resentment, Karen realized that injustice was merely a fabrication of her mind. An enormous weight seemed to slide from her shoulders. For the first time in months, she felt completely relaxed and free of muscular tension.

In the days that followed, Karen's arthritis pain gradually subsided. She did have two more mild flare-ups. But each time the pain was briefer and less intense. The last flare-up occurred two years later and Karen hasn't felt a twinge of pain or inflammation since. What happened, of course, is that as soon as Karen transformed her unforgiveness into

352

forgiveness, normality returned to her immune system and her arthritis vanished.

Nowadays, as soon as she experiences any type of conflict or stress, Karen completely forgives the person concerned. She simply witnesses the event without making any judgments and without becoming emotionally involved. By not becoming upset, she is better able to solve the conflict.

Karen is well aware the her new beliefs and values are not currently embraced by our money-driven culture. In today's competitive society, forgiving someone is often considered a sign of weakness. People seek revenge instead.

But letting go of a grudge can provide a powerful boost to your immunity. According to Redford Williams, M.D., psychiatrist and director of the behavioral research center at Duke University, chronic feelings of hostility actually assault the immune system.

The literature is filled with examples of people who have sought revenge on a relative, other person or even a corporation and who have been stricken with cancer, pneumonia or some other lethal disease. The emotional fallout from hostile beliefs and feelings can suppress the immune system, allowing cancer and a host of other diseases to appear in the body.

How to Get Rid of Counterproductive Beliefs from the Past

While unforgiveness is probably responsible for more immuno-suppression than any other negative belief, most of us have at least a dozen other immune-damaging beliefs in our minds. Knowing what they are isn't really important.

Key to success is knowing the new, positive beliefs you

want to adopt instead. As you install each new, positive belief in your mind, it will overlay and annul the negative belief that is suppressing your immunity. In any event, the Zen technique will help you identify and get rid of whatever negative beliefs are suppressing your immune system.

Most positive beliefs are framed as affirmations. To minimize stress and depression, I recommend adopting some or all of the 10 groups of affirmations listed below. As you read them, you may recognize that you hold an opposing viewpoint or belief. If you feel constantly stressed, anxious or depressed, you will undoubtedly benefit from letting go of the negative belief that is responsible for it and replacing it with a diametrically different, positive affirmation. Use the Zen technique and reprogram only one belief at a time.

THE TEN MOST POWERFUL IMMUNE-BOOSTING BELIEFS

1. I relieve all stress and depression—and I boost my immunity—as I let go of fear and replace it with unconditional love. I love everyone unconditionally and most especially myself. I accept everyone the way they are without requiring them to change.

2. I recognize that lasting happiness and fulfillment come only from being content and not from things I do, buy, eat or drink. Thus I do and acquire only things that will maintain and deepen my inner peace. I cease craving superficial excitement and stimulation. When I am content and at ease, my body-mind is calm, centered and relaxed. Thus I make choices and decisions only when I am calm and relaxed.

3. I know that absolute security is unobtainable. I always

354

have everything I need to enjoy the present moment. Thus my needs and wants are few. Excluding my occupation, I never expect a reward for my actions. I never seek fame, praise or recognition, and I refuse to do anything to win another person's approval. I also recognize that giving and receiving are the same. Whatever I give away or lose, I will receive back several times over. (Note that this does not apply to gambling, betting, "loaning" money to a financially irresponsible person, including a member of your own family, or giving away money of any amount without careful consideration.)

4. I can only win when everyone wins. Therefore I think in terms of cooperation rather than competition. Instead of competing, I will relax and enjoy every moment of every day regardless of where I am, who I'm with, how I'm feeling or what I'm doing. To free myself from envy, I avoid comparing myself with others or with their possessions or accomplishments; and I am willing to celebrate the good and the success achieved by others without feeling jealous.

5. I see each problem as a challenge and as a fresh opportunity to progress, grow and learn and not as a fight against the clock, another person or corporation. I accept complete responsibility for who I am, for everything I do and for almost everything that happens to me.

6. I realize that time does not heal wounds unless I actively forgive. Thus I forgive and release anyone I have not forgiven, including myself. I forgive everyone, everything and every circumstance totally and right now. Nor do I expect to be treated with justice and fairness. I realize that these are merely qualities in my mind, and I am ready to forgive anyone whom my mind perceives as unfair or unjust.

7. Whether in thought, word or deed, I cease to judge, criticize or condemn another person. I see only the best in

355

everyone, including and most especially myself. I experience a profound oneness with other people, and I refuse to see myself as separate or different. Whenever I meet another person, I look for the similarities between us rather than the differences.

8. I have totally ceased to worry about the future. All my fears about the future exist only in my imagination. I am a powerful person, and I am completely capable of handling whatever the future may bring. Besides, when the future arrives, it will have become the present. I also totally let go of the past and with it all guilt and resentment.

9. I am always optimistic, hopeful, cheerful and positive. I expect good things to happen to me today, tomorrow and throughout life. I recognize that to exist is bliss, to be here is joy and to be alive is pure happiness. Joy and bliss are my birthright, and I can experience them endlessly unless I permit a fear-based belief to influence my thoughts.

10. My birthright is perfect health, protected by a vigorous immune system—plus freedom from depression, cancer and infections. Perfect health is my normal, natural state. To achieve it, I am willing to use my mind and muscles to do whatever it takes to succeed. I am never intimidated by any minor discomfort or inconvenience nor by mental or physical exertion. Above all, I always act as if it is impossible to fail.

Affirmations like these may seem out of place in a society in which violence and revenge are the theme of hundreds of books, movies and TV shows each week. But these basic principles of wisdom are as effective today as they were 2,000 to 4,000 years ago when they were first discovered by ancient sages.

Despite all the stress, crime, drugs, isolation and the intolerable pace of life in modern society, when you analyze the reason for the stress and depression in your life, you will find that most is caused by perceiving the world through beliefs which are the very opposite of those in the affirmations just listed.

The choice is up to you.

You can choose to embrace the belief and value system of our aggressive, angry, competitive and violent society and go on suffering and popping pills. Or you can choose to make a complete paradigm shift and adopt a positive belief system that can send your immune system soaring.

To do this, practice the Zen temple technique. Use it to discover the most destructive negative belief that is causing stress and depression in your life. Then, in the same visualization, replace it with an opposite, but strongly positive belief from the affirmations just given.

Repeat the visualization once each day for a week. When you feel confident that the belief has been replaced, use the same technique to identify your second most destructive belief. Replace that, too, with a diametrically opposite, positive belief. Then keep on reprogramming one negative belief each week.

As well as using the Zen temple imagery, you can repeat the new, positive affirmation to yourself at intervals during the day. All this may not be quite as simple as swallowing a dietary supplement. But when it comes to boosting your immunity, cognitive positivism can be a 100 times more effective.

365